Leabharlanna Poiblí Átha Cliath
Dublin Public Libraries

Books should be returned on or before the last date shown below.
Books (not already requested by other borrowers) may be renewed by personal
application, by writing, or by telephone.

Borrowers' tickets may be used in any of the Dublin Municipal Libraries.

Damage to or loss of books will be charged to the borrower.

Borrowers must notify change of address.

Fines charged for overdue books will include postage incurred in recovery.

D1440402

Spina Bifida

The Treatment and Care of Spina Bifida Children

NANCY ALLUM

London   George Allen & Unwin Ltd
Ruskin House   Museum Street

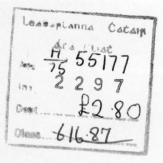

Printed in Great Britain
in 11 point Times Roman type
by Clarke, Doble & Brendon Ltd
Plymouth

My baby has not lived in vain – this life has been to him what it is to all of us, education and development.

Samuel Taylor Coleridge
(Letter to Thomas Poole, 6 April 1799)

THIS BOOK IS DEDICATED TO THE PARENTS

Preface

'If we know what we must cope with, we can cope.' These words spoken by a parent of a severely handicapped spina bifida child are characteristic of the courageous and undramatic way in which many spina bifida parents face their difficulties.

I have written *Spina Bifida* under the close guidance of a group of spina bifida specialists and the medical views given are those expressed by the team working in the Welsh National School of Medicine. The aim of this book is to show the parents of a new baby born with this handicap that they are not alone in their struggle. A further aim is to show what the problems are and how some of them can be alleviated.

By showing friends, neighbours and the general public what is involved in raising a spina bifida child, I hope that understanding and sympathy will be increased and that more assistance on a personal level, and perhaps on a much larger scale also, will result. That is one of the reasons why the families interviewed for these pages have co-operated so wholeheartedly in talking to me about their lives, their difficulties and their achievements, and in allowing their photographs to be used.

I have stressed the need of every handicapped child for access to a good school, with a suitable routine for his handicap. This is needed not only for the sake of the child and the family but, in the long run, for the sake of the community. Wherever possible the family should be relieved of unnecessary stress, and whatever burdens they must bear should be lightened by being shared, so that we do not end up with overstrained parents, broken families and destroyed marriages.

But one of the dangers in writing about spina bifida

cystica and hydrocephalus, or any other medical problem for that matter, is that parents may suppose their child will have all the problems that are discussed. For this reason I want to repeat what the specialist social worker who guided me in the family interviews has always emphasised – 'Every spina bifida baby is different.' Ideally every child should have a separate book for his parents' guidance. But that is not possible and in any case, as is well known, parents soon become the experts about their own child.

Much help is available for the handicapped in the United Kingdom. Not everyone is aware of this fact. When The Chronically Sick and Disabled Persons Act 1970 was before Parliament, the need was stressed for greater publicity about the help available to the handicapped and their families. With these objects in view I hope this book will help as many parents as possible, from those whose child needs hardly any extra assistance at all to those whose child is very severely handicapped indeed.

I am deeply grateful for all the help and encouragement I have received from the Cardiff team which, when this book was started, consisted of: E. H. Hare, M.D., K. M. Laurence, M.A., M.B., Ch.B., F.R.C. Path., E. R. Laurence, B.A., Helly Payne, Research Social Worker, K. Rawnsley, M.B., Ch.B., F.R.C.P., D.P.M., and Brian Tew, B.A., Dip. Psych. A.B.Ps.S.

I am also most grateful to Dr M. Thomas for her advice on the urinary problems of spina bifida children, and to Mrs Weber for her instruction on physiotherapy. I wish to thank, too, all the teachers and nurses who gave me helpful guidance.

Specially among the Cardiff group, however, Dr Laurence and the specialist social worker Mrs Helly Payne have given their time unstintingly. I am also particularly indebted to Dr Hare who persuaded me to become involved in the subject. If this book does manage to bring some help and comfort to the families, it is very largely due to the assistance of these dedicated workers in the field of spina bifida.

I am indebted to Mr Ralph Marshall of the Department

of Medical Illustration of the Welsh National School of Medicine for the use of his photographs and to Thomson Newspapers of Cardiff for the photograph of the Holiday Home. I am also indebted to Mr T. J. Cooke, Department of Child Health, the Welsh School of Medicine, for the diagrams.

Nancy Allum
September 1974

Contents

There are photographs between pages 32 and 33 and 48 and 49.

Chapter 1

What is Spina Bifida?

The birth of a baby is always a tremendous event. For some parents the joy of this moment of birth is turned to distress by the news that their baby has 'spina bifida' and by the warning that he will probably be physically handicapped. The event is made even more distressing by the fact that the baby will probably have to be taken away from the mother and operated on as soon as possible after birth in order to give him the best chance for his life later on.

The words 'spina bifida', Latin words which mean 'spine split in two', do not give an accurate description of what the condition is but they are used to give a name to a group of congenital malformations of the central nervous system. Spina bifida cystica is one of the major crippling disorders in this country. About 1,500 children are born with the condition each year in England and Wales, approximately a quarter of them being stillborn. After mental retardation it is the most frequent in occurrence and has overtaken cerebral palsy in this respect.

The condition has probably always been with us. Its existence has been documented since the seventeenth century and was well known to physicians many centuries before that. Up to a decade or so ago few children with spina bifida survived because they died from meningitis or the effects of untreated *hydrocephalus* and many who did survive were so handicapped they had to be cared for in long-stay institutions. Nowadays, with modern treatment and care, some of the complications can be alleviated and more than half the children survive into school life and beyond. The incidence of this malformation in the United

Kingdom is 2·4 per thousand births. In other parts of the world the incidence seems to be lower.

How does it happen that a child is born with spina bifida?

In the normally developing human embryo the part that develops into the central nervous system begins as a sheet of cells which curls back on itself to, form a tube. The closure of the tube should be completed by the end of the fourth week after conception. At the same time the *meninges* (from the Greek for 'covering'), the spinal column and the skull are being formed from another group of cells.

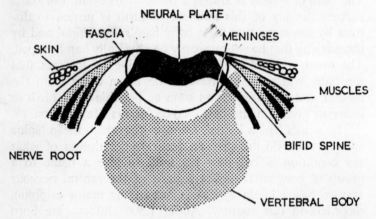

Diagrammatic view of a cross-section of a myelocele.

When something goes wrong with the lower end of this tube which is destined to become the spinal cord, spina bifida in any of its various forms may result. When something goes wrong with this process at the top end of the tube destined to become the brain, the abnormality known as 'anencephaly' (from a Greek word meaning 'without brain') results. This is a condition in which the head is not developed properly. Anencephaly occurs almost as often as spina bifida but it is incompatible with life.

Spina bifida may be of two kinds. It may be 'cystica' (cystlike), or 'occulta' which means hidden. This second kind of spina bifida is very common, it is found in 10 per cent of the population and is the least serious. There may be no external evidence of its presence, or there may be abnormality of the skin such as a birthmark, or a patch of hair, or a mere dimple. It is rarely accompanied by any form of disability and is therefore usually of no great significance.

Spina bifida cystica is always obvious at birth. This malformation is divided into two main types. In the less serious type only the meninges bulge through the gap in

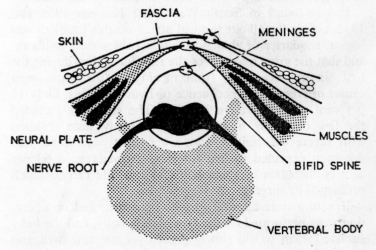

FASCIA

SKIN

MENINGES

NEURAL PLATE

MUSCLES

NERVE ROOT

BIFID SPINE

VERTEBRAL BODY

Diagrammatic view of a cross-section of a repaired myelocele with meninges and facia as well as skin brought over the neural tissue.

the spine and the resulting abnormality is called a *'meningocele'* (from the Greek words meaning 'a bulge in the coverings'). It is relatively uncommon, and as the brain and spinal cord are usually normal there is generally no paralysis, incontinence or hydrocephalus. The area of damage is often referred to as the *'lesion'*.

The much more common type of spina bifida cystica occurs when the tissue of the spinal cord forms part of the cystic swelling or lies exposed on the surface of the back when the baby is born. This form is called the *'myelomeningocele'* or the *'myelocele'*. (The Greek word myelos means pith or marrow and in medicine refers to the spinal cord.)

The most severe cases usually have visible *hydrocephalus*, Greek for 'water on the brain') as well; and almost all are associated with paralysis of the legs, incontinence and often deformity of the feet. In less severe cases paralysis and incontinence may be partial, and the hydrocephalus may be minimal. Sometimes a myelomeningocele causes only minor nerve involvement, resulting in very little disability. The term 'encephalocele' is used for a type of spina bifida occurring at the top of the neck or back of the head.

It was found in South Wales that between 1956 and 1962, before the all-out surgical attack on this problem was begun, a quarter of the spina bifida babies were stillborn, and that the great majority of the remainder died during the first six months either from meningitis (the commonest cause) or from the consequence of hydrocephalus. Only 15 per cent were still alive in 1971. The survivors included the few obviously milder cases but many were children with severe deformities who, when they were born, had not been expected to live for long. Nowadays, in 60 per cent of the cases of spina bifida cystica, life can be much prolonged by surgery.

If nature were allowed to take its course and no operation were performed on the spina bifida baby, and the baby survived, skin would slowly grow over the raw area and would eventually protect the nerve tissue to a certain extent but in the process a lot of damage would occur. Moreover this skin tends to be papery; it is easily damaged and that may sometimes lead to meningitis. Every effort has to be made to avoid this since meningitis commonly causes damage to the brain, and later a loss of learning ability. Nowadays an operation is often performed to protect the nerve tissue and reduce the incidence of local infection and of meningitis.

These are the steps generally taken once it is realised by whoever is attending the birth that a baby has spina bifida cystica. If a malformation is present the midwife has to call the doctor. When the midwife and doctor see the problem, they telephone the hospital for the baby to be taken in immediately to find out if an operation is necessary and can be performed. In most cases the child is sent to a specialised spina bifida centre. If an operation is decided on, the mother and baby are separated for about two or more weeks, but during this time the mother is generally able to visit the baby and learn how to manage him when she takes him home.

When the baby is in hospital, usually within twenty-four hours of birth but anyway as soon as possible, the baby is examined by a surgeon. If he decides that an operation is indicated, his aim will be to cover the raw, exposed spinal cord tissue with a full-thickness skin. Sometimes he will remove some of the redundant membrane and refashion the spinal cord and its covering as well as possible. The exact course of the operation depends on what the surgeon finds when examining the baby on the operating table. The first aim is to preserve the healthy nerve tissue, and to prevent meningitis and further damage and loss of function. Since it is not possible to grow or to implant a new spinal cord, the surgeon can only help to preserve and protect what the child has.

The result of the closure operation depends on the original state of the spinal cord, on whether it was already infected and on whether the skin closure heals by 'first intention', in surgeon's language, that is without infection. After the operation some children are lucky and have no paralysis at all, others may have only slight weakness in a few muscles, but others may have little use of their muscles at all below the neurological level of the *lesion* in the spinal cord (the level that is controlled by the nerves that are involved in the paralysis).

Most spina bifida cystica babies are born with at least some degree of hydrocephalus. This may be present even if the head is not obviously enlarged. In some cases the hydrocephalus may not get worse and may arrest itself spontaneously, but in many others it gets progressively worse. If there are signs of the hydrocephalus increasing, a drainage operation is usually performed to divert the accumulating spinal fluid from the brain back into the blood stream or into one of the body cavities from which it will be

B

absorbed. Some surgeons operate on the head before they repair the back, but most deal with the back first and then, as soon as things have settled down, deal with the hydrocephalus if necessary.

There are a number of different drainage operations in common use. Nearly all take the form of inserting a tube with some sort of non-return valve so that the fluid in the head returns to the circulation, usually by way of a valve leading into the heart. In one of the techniques the valve is placed under the skin behind the ear and in others the valve is in a different position. The valve may become blocked by a clot or by debris and it may become infected since any foreign body may become the centre for the growth of harmful bacteria. Thus there is a tendency for chronic low-grade infection to occur, which may cause abscesses or kidney trouble, a tendency which has to be fought with constant vigilance by parents and the medical team.

Sometimes the infection can be dealt with by massive dosing with antibiotics but often the valve has to be removed and another one inserted. Some children have to have the valve replaced several times. The valve insertion and the valve changes are not big operations but they are vitally important. After the valve has been inserted the abnormal rate of the head expansion is stopped, the scars soon heal and disappear and no one would know the valve was there. Careful measurements of the head are made regularly by the hospitals to check that all goes well. Some of the operations draining the fluid into the body cavities often do not require a valve as part of the draining system, but they are sometimes associated with other problems.

The story of one valve's invention and its first use is a moving one. A spina bifida baby girl was born to an American fluids engineer named Holter and his wife. When the little girl, whose name was Casey, developed hydrocephalus the parents took her to a surgeon in Philadelphia. The surgeon in charge of the case said he was sorry there was nothing he could do for the child because his hospital had no suitable valve with which to draw off the cerebro-spinal fluid. 'If you can invent a valve which will work', he told the fluids engineer, 'we can insert it.'

Mr Holter went back and invented one in a matter of days. His daughter was given a modified version of it. Casey Holter's life was prolonged by the invention, but she died when she was four years old and a lecture in her memory is given every two years by a selected prominent worker in the field of hydrocephalus. The valve used for Casey Holter, which has been improved over the years, is the type that is used most in this country and probably throughout the

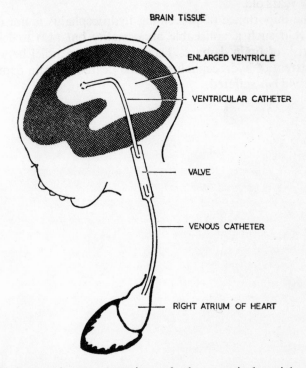

Diagrammatic representation of the ventriculo-atrial shunt (Holter) operation. The ventricular catheter lies in the dilated cerebral ventricle. The valve housing lies on the skull behind the ear and the cardiac catheter is brought through a large vein into the right atrial chamber of the heart.

world. It has been of enormous benefit to thousands of children who would otherwise have had to suffer from the further effects of hydrocephalus.

Parents of a baby who has first had a valve inserted can derive comfort from the fact that even if the baby's head has become enlarged, insertion of the valve having stopped the abnormal growth rate, the baby's body will grow fast and in most cases will soon, in about two years, match the head size, and the hydrocephalus will no longer be obvious to the ordinary observer. There are many photographs in existence which show how an infant whose head was obviously oversized in babyhood had grown to 'fit it' when the baby was a few years old.

The importance of preventing hydrocephalus is not only to avoid such a noticeable abnormality but also to lessen the risk of brain damage. There is a close parallel between the extent of hydrocephalus and the degree of brain damage the child has suffered.

Chapter 2

What are the Causes of Spina Bifida?

It is a tragic and surprising fact that the death rate from congenital malformations has not been affected by the rise in the standard of living that has taken place in technically advanced countries. In England and Wales infant deaths certified as due to congenital malformations have remained at four to five in a thousand since the turn of the century, while total infant mortality has gone down dramatically from 130 to 20 in 1,000 births.[1]

The position in the rest of the world is hard to discover with any accuracy since some countries are very poor in statistical data and others record their facts in a different way from that used in the United Kingdom. For instance we can tell from the World Health Organisation reports[1] that in some countries (for example in Poland), the newborn are recorded as 'live' only if they survive the first twenty-four hours; in other countries they are recorded as 'live' if they are still alive when the birth is officially registered. This is the case, for instance, in Algeria, France, Greece, Luxembourg, Morocco and Spain. This practice makes the number of late foetal deaths higher in relation to deaths just after birth than they would appear if they were recorded as in this country.

Another point to take into consideration is that in some countries such as Bulgaria and Rumania they have fairly low perinatal[2] mortality rates, although the late infant mor-

[1] 'The prevention of perinatal morbidity and mortality', Public Health Papers (42) WHO Geneva.
[2] There are different interpretations of this term. In the U.K. 'perinatal' means 'at birth and up to seven days after birth'.

tality rate there is still quite high. These countries practice or have practised interruption of pregnancy on a large scale. As many such abortions are authorised for medical reasons such as poor health, advancing age of the mother and so on, they probably eliminate births that would later have been particularly at risk.

These are just a few of the problems that make true comparisons difficult on an international basis, and they illustrate the danger of basing too many conclusions on statistics, the origins of which have not been carefully weighed and compared.

Early detection of severe foetal malformation and termination of pregnancy have been practised in the United Kingdom for some time. Anencephaly and hydrocephalus, for instance, can be detected by scanning the baby in the womb with ultrasonic waves which bounce back off the baby. These waves can be recorded in a way that will show whether either of these conditions is present. Ultrasonic examination carries no risk for mother or for the baby so far as is known. The examination can be carried out as early as the twelfth week and is usually repeated a month or so later. Spina bifida itself cannot at the moment be detected in this way.

However, a test is now available for doing this. In this process, at about four months after conception, some fluid from the womb is examined for an abnormal constituent which gets into the womb fluid, having seeped out through an exposed spina bifida. This test is successful in detecting nearly all cases of anencephaly and most, if not all, cases of spina bifida. It is of minimal risk to mother and baby though occasionally it may cause a miscarriage. Because of this it should only be used when there is a high risk of abnormality such as there is when a mother has already had a malformed baby. The substance being sought by the laboratories in this test is a protein which is normally confined to the foetus but which in the presence of an exposed spina bifida can seep into the amniotic fluid (the fluid in the womb). The technique of extracting fluid from the womb is called "amniocentesis'.

Because of the risks to mother and baby of X-ray examination, this method is generally avoided unless there is very strong indication that there is something wrong with the baby or the mother. One of the indications of such a risk is the accumulation of too much fluid. This happens, for instance, with anencephaly. Another reason why X-rays are not used to try to detect spina bifida is that it is very difficult to identify the condition in time, as the bones do not show until about the twenty-third or twenty-fourth week, and termination of pregnancy, if necessary, should be done before the twentieth week. A further difficulty is that spina bifida is not readily revealed in an X-ray unless the baby is in a very favourable position in the womb, or unless there is a malpositioning of the limbs or spine, and this will only be apparent when it is too late to terminate the pregnancy.

What are the causes of spina bifida? Anyone who could answer this question with certainty would be one of the benefactors of mankind since if the cause were known steps could be taken to attack the problem at source. Certain facts are known. The condition exists in the foetus as early as five weeks after conception. The cause is thought to be a combination of genetic influences and environmental influences such as, for instance, the water supply, diet or minor infections; but none of these particular environmental influences has been proved to be responsible.

Blighted potatoes have been the subject of much scrutiny recently. It was noticed that in some areas of the world a high incidence of neural tube malformations coincided with a high incidence of potato blight. Some researchers believed that *solanaceous alkaloids* in blighted potatoes caused the vast majority of cases of neural tube malformations, and that potato avoidance in early pregnancy would eliminate most cases of spina bifida. The hard evidence for this is slender, and there is a great deal of evidence to suggest in fact that potato blight is not a major causal factor in the occurrence. For example there is a high incidence of spina bifida in Taiwan; but the only people there who eat potatoes are Europeans and they have a low incidence.

Since the water supply has been questioned, as a result of some studies, it can now be said that there is probably some sort of association between soft water and spina bifida. There is some suggestion that whatever factor is responsible for the association is not responsible for the increase in the number of cases being conceived, but for an increase in the number of babies being retained in the uterus. There is quite a lot of evidence that the number of spina bifida and anencephalic conceptions is bigger than the number of such births. In a considerable proportion of miscarriages the foetus is already malformed and abnormal.

As has already been pointed out, conclusions based on available statistics, particularly from world statistics of infant deaths, have to be regarded with suspicion. Even in a country as technologically developed as Great Britain it used to be the custom not to tell the mother of a stillborn baby that her child had had spina bifida, or even that it had been malformed at all. Even in the realms of fiction it is hard to recall any cases where there is a description or even an allusion to a malformed baby. The child is generally termed 'sickly', 'weak' or just 'stillborn'. The rest is a romantic silence. No doubt this mystery and secrecy is continued in real life in many communities today and where this is so, such births are obviously not going to be recorded in their correct category for statistical purposes.

However, while the search for the cause of these malformations goes on we are forced to use statistics as the best evidence available, and from the ones presented it appears race is certainly a relevant factor since there is considerable variation of their incidence in different parts of the world. For example, the incidence in South Wales and Northern Ireland is particularly high, much higher than in the rest of the United Kingdom. Again, a study carried out in Boston, North America, showed babies born to parents of Irish origin in the city had a much higher incidence than those of Jewish origin. The incidence among Negroes is very low. There are also marked rises and falls of incidence from year to year in the areas studied.

The evidence shows there is a greater incidence among firstborn children and among the offspring of the youngest and the oldest group of mothers. The father's age appears to have no independent effect. More female than male children are affected and there is a higher incidence in the lower socio-economic classes.

At a time when most of us have ceased to think in terms of social classes the sociologists seem to employ such classifications more and more. However, the fact is that statistics have been repeatedly produced which point to spina bifida hitting hardest the lower socio-economic groups. In a sense it is true that all such problems hit the lower socio-economic groups hardest to the extent that the mothers who are short of money, time, and probably energy, often do not have the resources and the stamina to go through the processes of seeking help in family planning or genetic counselling or make use of the other social services available, or even to feed themselves properly. But is there a closer connection than that between spina bifida and the social classification?

Apart from cases where there is exceptional hardship, it is hard to see any difference in the physical lives of the mothers in the various socio-economic classes that might affect an embryo baby, and this is true whether we are thinking in terms of eating, drinking or the use of pharmaceutical products. Furthermore, many spina bifida babies come from very comfortable, well-run homes where there is no important material shortage, whatever the socio-economic grouping of the parents.

Geneticists believe there is a hereditary factor in spina bifida but that there must also be environmental or other factors because its incidence is not nearly as high as would be expected if it were a purely hereditary condition. It is thought that quite minor metabolic disturbances, deficiencies or infections, within twenty-eight days of conception, could be the cause.

Causes of malformations of the central nervous system are one of the spheres in which much can be hoped for from research and this work is being carried out as a matter of urgency by many organisations, both official and private. Official support for medical research in the United Kingdom is provided through three main and complementary sources – the universities, the National Health Service and the

Medical Research Council. In addition to the official support of medical research, an important contribution is made by private foundations and charitable organisations in this country and abroad, several of which concern themselves with the handicaps of children.

In the United Kingdom the Children's Research Fund supports research into all children's diseases and allocates some £150,000 a year in grants to child health research centres. The Mental Health Research Fund supports all types and fields of mental research. A large sum is allocated by them annually in fellowships and grants. The National Fund for Research into Crippling Diseases was founded in 1952 as the National Fund for Poliomyelitis Research, changing to the present title in 1966. It is heartening to reflect that because of progress in fighting poliomyelitis its resources are now distributed over a wider field of research into the causes, cure and alleviation of effects of diseases and congenital defects which cripple, with particular emphasis on children. The National Society for Mentally Handicapped Children allocates funds to research on the advice of the Institute for Research into Mental Retardation. The Nuffield Provincial Hospitals Trust contributes handsomely to medical research of all kinds. The Association for Spina Bifida and Hydrocephalus promotes research into the treatment, causes and prevention of spina bifida and hydrocephalus and gives support to those born with these handicaps. (Some information about its research programmes is given at the end of this book.)

There are many more organisations which make contributions to medical research. One of special interest in the South Wales area is 'Tenovus', an organisation founded in 1943 by ten Cardiff businessmen. Tenovus became an established institution, raising funds for many purposes over a wide area. Because the prevalence of spina bifida is particularly high in South Wales (it rises to over 6·5 per thousand births in certain parts compared with the average of about 2·6 per thousand for the whole of the British Isles) they have provided a special ward for the treatment and nursing of spina bifida children – the first in the world.

Between seventy and eighty new children a year are now being treated in this unit.

Tenovus have also set up a research project in mass spectrometry which will make possible the measurement of extremely small quantities of elements in blood, water, soil, tissue, body fluids and so on. Using this new technique and working closely with other disciplines, they are making a concentrated effort to discover what it is that upsets the normal growth of a baby. They are trying to answer the questions: 'Why should any child be born with spina bifida?' and 'Why are so many in South Wales so stricken?'

Official support for medical research in Scotland is available from the Medical Research Council, the Research Subhead of the National Health Service (Scotland) Vote, the Regional Hospital Board research funds, the Board of Management endowment funds, and the Scottish Hospital Endowments Research Trust.

In the United States of America spina bifida is not reportable so the Department of Health, Education and Welfare has no accurate information as to how many cases occur, but an estimate of 11,000 new cases a year is suggested. However, a great deal of research into spina bifida and hydrocephalus and other disorders of the developing nervous system, is being carried out in certain universities there, and The National Institute of Neurological Diseases and Stroke (NINDS), conducts and supports research on neurological disorders of early life, including spina bifida, to the tune of about $13,000,000 a year.

Since 1959 the Collaborative Perinatal Study has monitored a total of 55,908 women and their pregnancies, in search of relationships between factors occurring during the perinatal period (in the United States this term means 'from conception to 28 days after birth') and a child's neurological development. During 1972 an important milestone in the progress of this analysis was the publication of *The Women and Their Pregnancies*, a broad review of the nature and scope of the associations found among the Study data. The book details the Study design, population, procedures, protocol and data processing used, and also ex-

plains the characteristics of the abnormal conditions,
environmental factors, and biological factors of the pregnancies studied, and shows their possible relationships to
favourable and unfavourable outcomes.

There is much voluntary activity too in the United States.
For instance the Association for the Aid of Crippled
Children, founded in 1900, allocates approximately a million
US dollars a year to research for 'the advancement of knowledge and understanding of causes and consequences of
handicap, primarily in children'. This Association supports
research within the broad spectrum of developmental problems both pre- and post-natal, including investigations in
biomedical and behavioural science.

*(The addresses of the various organisations supporting
research mentioned in this chapter are given at the end of
this book.)*

Chapter 3

Help from the Medical Team

What are the special needs of the child with spina bifida? A lot of time has to be spent on him in order to deal with his physical needs alone and yet parents have to try to treat him normally and not give him the impression he is more important or more powerful than the other members of the family. This is one of the recommendations that are so easy for the outsider to make and so hard for the parents to carry out. It is even hard for parents to assess whether they are spoiling their handicapped child or not. This is an important matter since it has been found that the normal brothers and sisters of severely handicapped spina bifida children sometimes show maladjustment which was probably brought on by the disproportionate amount of time and energy that had to be given to the handicapped child.

The handicapped child should be trained for a place in the community by being taught consideration for others, good manners and good eating habits. For instance he should be shown how to use a knife and fork at the same stage as any normal child.

Other areas of his home education that will help him fit into society are learning to dress and undress himself, even if this takes a long time at first. He should be taught to wash his hands and face, clean his teeth, comb his hair and blow his nose. These matters seem obvious but some parents are so anxious to help, or in some cases the children are so demanding, that these small tasks sometimes get done for them even when they are perfectly capable of doing them for themselves. Not only that, it is often quicker for the mother to do them herself.

The handicapped child should often be read to and encouraged to join in discussions about the stories and pictures in the book. He should be taught to widen his vocabulary, practise counting, to sort out cutlery, buttons, clothes and so on. He should be taught a few small jobs about the home too. He can learn games and he should play them with other children as much as possible to help him to adapt to his own generation. When he is playing with other children parents should not interfere if their handicapped child does not always get his own way.

Children love playing with sand and water, dough, plasticine, bricks, and graded beakers. They enjoy playing 'houses', dressing and undressing dolls, laying a doll's table, sticking and gluing things, paper tearing, using scissors, doing simple jigsaws, playing games such as 'Snap', 'Snakes and Ladders', 'Lotto' and so on. And of course it is excellent for the handicapped child's morale if he can become expert in some game of mental skill such as dominoes or draughts.

Another way in which children with spina bifida can be helped is by watching their weight. Life is made harder for them if they are allowed to get fat. This often happens, and for three reasons. First of all, as they are physically handicapped they are less active than normal children. (The less active person tends to put on weight because he does not use up his food intake.) Secondly, because they are less active they have more time to eat and think about food. Thirdly, parents tend to overfeed their child, often because they are trying to make up for his handicap. It is a self-aggravating problem since the bigger you get the less mobile you become and so on. The spina bifida child should be given an interesting and varied diet but he should be served small helpings – a fact that may have to be explained to him!

Skill and patience are needed to deal with incontinence to stop it becoming a major problem for some children with spina bifida. What is the cause of this trouble? In the normal body two kidneys filter the waste products from the blood stream and the resultant liquid, urine, then passes down through two elastic tubes known as *'ureters'* into the bladder. As the bladder fills, the physically normal person receives 'messages' in the form of feelings, to which he can react by controlling his bladder muscles and forcing out the urine. The amount of force required depends on the tightness of the *sphincter* muscle at the exit point of the bladder. The urine flows out through a single tube, the urethra. In the female the urethra ends just above the vagina, and in the male at the tip of the penis.

If for any reason the bladder is not under control it will stretch, the connecting ureters will fill up and they too will come under pressure. If this process is not halted the bladder and the ureters will become enlarged and lose their shape and elasticity. The enlargement of the ureters can compress the kidneys and damage them and impair the filtering mechanism. When this happens waste products are not filtered out but circulate through the body. When renal failure occurs vital organs may be damaged and this constitutes a real risk to life.

It sometimes happens too that the bladder stores the urine and only expels the overflow. If this occurs this condition must be dealt with as soon as possible since stagnant urine too is a source of dangerous infection.

All human bladders and rectums fill up and need emptying regularly. Most people with spina bifida cystica suffer from lack of control of the bowel and bladder. When considering the problems of incontinence in childhood, adolescence and adulthood, sad as the difficulty is and one not to be under-rated, it is still to be remembered that all normal people have to make arrangements to visit the lavatory and quite a few have occasional discomfort or find themselves in an embarrassing situation from time to time. This may seem a needless observation but sometimes the fact does seem to be lost sight of when the incontinence of some handicapped people is discussed.

Parents of spina bifida babies can help their children from the earliest days by training them to help themselves as much as possible in matters of excretion. Paediatricians and physiotherapists have some guidance to give in this respect. The more children who are incontinent can achieve in this direction, the more easily acceptable they will be to general society. With skill, care and perseverance, many children and adults with spina bifida involving some incontinence finally manage to cope so well with these difficulties that others are unaware of their problems.

Mothers are advised to start training their children from the age of one month by potting them regularly. To encourage bowel movement the baby should be held in a squatting position. He should be supported until he is able to sit safely on the pot on his own. It is generally found easier to hold the baby from behind with the adult also sitting. The baby's feet should be firmly on the floor and not dangling.

Various tricks and games may be suggested to give the child the right idea, tricks such as asking him to blow up a balloon, making him pretend to cough or making him laugh. Some children 'go' regularly after every meal and some 'go' once a day. Other recommendations to help the child have regular bowel movements are adding bran to the diet and regulating the amount of fruit eaten to suit the needs of the particular child. Suppositories inserted in the rectum are also helpful but their size has to be carefully adjusted to the child. Rectal plugs, sometimes useful for the elderly, are not considered suitable for the young.

Parents and the medical team have to steer a careful course to avoid the two extremes of constipation and diarrhoea. Purges are not suitable for handicapped children unless recommended by the doctor. This is another aspect in which it becomes clear that every spina bifida baby is different.

Self-confidence is a help with this problem. Some children know when they need to go to the lavatory but not having been trained when young are too shy to say what they want. A child with spina bifida who has been encouraged from his earliest moments to give some indication of his toilet needs is not shy about this. Most children with spina bifida can be trained to deal with faecal incontinence and develop an automatic bowel action once a day. On the

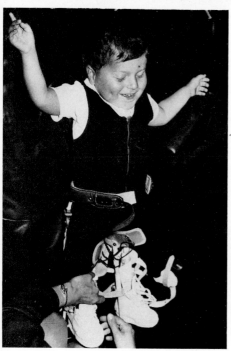

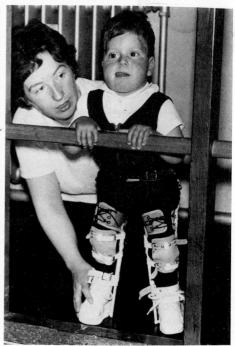

1. Nigel, aged four. Putting on calipers.

2. Nigel, calipers on and standing at the bar.

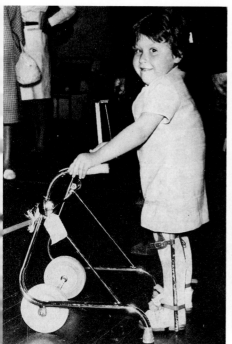

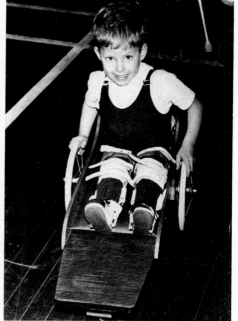

3. Sharon, with calipers and rolater.

4. Huw, aged four, very severely handicapped, mentally alert, enjoying a ride on his trolley.

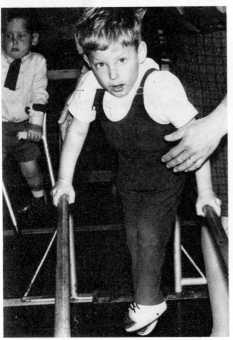

5. Huw, with his physiotherapist at the parallel bars.

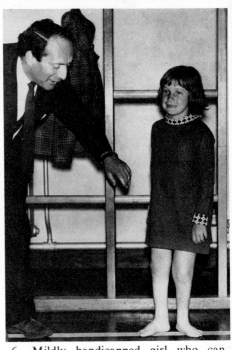

6. Mildly handicapped girl who can walk being aided by Dr Laurence.

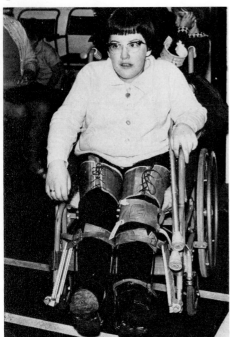

7. Janice with wheelchair, calipers and crutches. Wheelchair is used for longer distances and sitting comfort. For shorter distances Janice could manage with crutches and calipers.

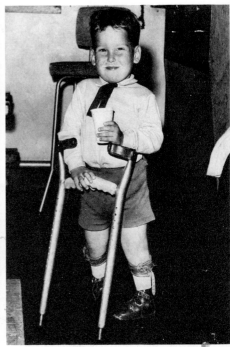

8. Russel in short leg irons. He is slightly hydrocephalic.

whole parents and medical teams find that bowel control is easier to achieve than urinary control.

What can be done to help in this direction? The condition of the spina bifida baby's renal system is examined as early as possible in his life and checks are continued at regular intervals. Parents are shown how to look out for signs of trouble. Urine should be clear in appearance. If it becomes thick, cloudy or smelly, medical help should be sought immediately. Feverishness and querulousness are often signs of urinary infection.

Regular and complete evacuation of the bladder at intervals of about two hours during the day should be aimed at and it is advisable to have urinary evacuation twice during the night. High fluid intake is of great assistance in attaining this and increasing the rate of urine formation diminishes the risk of infection from stagnant urine. It also helps to establish a routine. Antiseptic drugs are often prescribed by the doctor to help to avoid urinary infection. If the bladder is not being emptied every two hours evacuation should be encouraged by manual expression. This is done by applying gentle pressure over the bladder. This can be learnt by the parents, and many children soon learn to do it for themselves. Sometimes the sphincter muscle is too tight for evacuation even with manual assistance. In such cases the urological surgeon may decide to loosen the sphincter and to make manual evacuation easier and safer.

Girls have more complications than boys when it comes to the disposal of urine. Boys can often be kept dry for periods of one to three hours provided the bladder is expressed manually. Girls' urinary continence is much more difficult to achieve.

Sometimes an operation known as the 'ileal loop' operation is performed on girls. This involves diverting the urinary tract through a transplanted piece of intestine which is fashioned to form an outlet through the abdomen. This allows urine to be collected in a bag in the same way that it is for males. The outlet created by the operation is known as the 'stoma'. Many parents find the result unsightly and worrying but often young women with spina bifida prefer it to having to use nappies or other absorbent material. This operation is performed nowadays only if there is medical need, if the parents request it for their child, or if an adult requests it for herself. Sometimes, for therapeutic reasons the ileal loop operation is performed on boys.

With regard to appliances for urinary incontinence, the shape of the penis makes the collection of urine from the male much easier than from the female. The usual method is the wearing of a penile attachment and there are several types on the market. The ones selected should be comfortable, easy to adjust and keep clean, should not be too bulky and, obviously, should be effective. It is advisable to have at least three, and when choosing them to consider whether they are suitable for both night and day use, whether they are suitable for activity or inactivity and whether they are adaptable to social and working needs. They should be washed with soap and water and carefully dried on a rack.

Girls who have not had the 'bag' operation have to rely on absorbent pads of various kinds. The girls who have had the bag operation performed have special urine containers which should have the same qualities as those used by the boys. Some mothers have found difficulty in getting the girls' bags to remain in place.

Another aspect for girls that should be mentioned here is the possibility of the abnormally early onset of puberty; menstruation sometimes starts as early as eight years of age. Naturally parents and child should be psychologically prepared for this, the parents being warned by their doctor or health visitor and they in turn explaining matters to their daughter.

When considering the harm that may have been suffered by a child with spina bifida, the general guide is that damage caused by the spina bifida produces paralysis of the lower half of the body, and damage caused by any hydrocephalus that may have been present affects mental ability and co-ordination.

If a child seems slower than normal in his early mental development this may be due to his bad start, stays in hospital and so on, and if this is the only reason for it he will soon catch up as his life gets back to normal. But if he has suffered brain damage his progress will be slower.

Some children with spina bifida have to be medically checked regularly after the lump (the 'cystica') has been removed, the 'closure' or 'covering' operation has been completed, and the valve inserted, since after these processes there either may be almost negligible damage below the former lump or there may be partial or total paralysis.

The upper part of the trunk is generally normal but because the muscles of the lower part of the body may have varying degree of weakness, deformities may occur when the child assumes abnormal positions over a long period of time. An orthopaedic surgeon can often correct these deformities but the need for this can sometimes be avoided by exercises and physical therapy.

It sometimes happens that the hip joint is imperfect and nowadays orthopaedic surgeons deal with this early in the baby's life. Often the baby only needs to wear a special splint to hold the hip in the desired position for a short period and then the hip settles into its proper position. Sometimes, however, an operation is necessary.

If the feet are deformed they should be manipulated frequently from the earliest stages according to instructions given by specialists. After manipulation they are sometimes put into a plaster and this has to be changed at frequent intervals. In some cases the tendons of legs need to be lengthened, shortened or a transplant may need to be performed. In others the hips need manipulation and plasters, though these are being used less and less now that specialised tendon transplant operations are being successfully carried out.

The feet must be in a good position so that they can be used at least for support. A deformed foot is awkward to fit with shoes and is liable to develop pressure sores which may be difficult to treat. This is not only because the skin is liable to get hurt, as there is no feeling, but because skin without nerve tissue heals badly.

Aids such as splints, calipers, short-leg calipers, and

calipers right up to the hip to be used in conjunction with walking aids, help people with spina bifida to get around. For those for whom these aids are not of any use there are increasingly sophisticated wheel-chairs.

Since the range of needs varies so widely it is a help if parents can understand the whole concept of the programme of treatment for their child so that they, the medical team and the social workers can guide the child through the various stages, sharing the responsibility and appreciating the child's progress when things go well.

The parents should try to adopt the right attitude towards their child, being neither too gloomy nor too optimistic. I am well aware this is no easy matter as the parents sometimes find it takes all their energies to keep the family going and they may not have the additional stamina or patience to think too much about attitudes. However, they do need to achieve this realistic view both for their own sakes and their child's. This is precisely the sphere too in which the various supporting services can and do help but naturally they must be contacted by the family with the needs.

Education for the handicapped child is discussed in Chapter 6 but it should be said here that such children are helped by coming into contact with other children as early as possible and by attending school as early as possible. Since their education may be interrupted from time to time for the hospital check-ups and so on, they need to take advantage of every opportunity they can get to develop their social sense.

Chapter 4

Help from the Physiotherapists

Apart from the aid the medical team can give to a family with a spina bifida child, specialist welfare workers and health visitors can assist with advice, information and moral support. Physiotherapists, for instance, can do a lot to help the parents develop the baby's mental and physical potentialities so that he suffers as little deprivation as possible. They can help with the practical details of management at home as well as giving the baby treatment at the clinics. These are the sorts of treatment and attitudes recommended by a leading physiotherapist who has specialised in treating spina bifida children for many years.

The first priority is to cuddle and love the baby. It might seem superfluous to say this, but sometimes such a prime need of the baby gets overlooked. The mother of the handicapped baby does not always cuddle him as she would a normal child, perhaps through a feeling of fear she will hurt him, perhaps through a feeling of failure and perhaps because she does not want to become too fond of a baby she feels she may lose.

Then there is the need to help the baby get to know his physical world. Babies enjoy exploring their surroundings. They enjoy feeling them, smelling them and, as most have learned with a sudden shock, tasting them. Some handicapped babies need help in this adventure of exploring. Just because the child is quiet and good, he should not be left lying in his cot all day. He should be given every opportunity of following the normal sequence of his development, especially in the first months after birth.

The spina bifida baby with paralysed legs who may be

unable to move easily himself, needs to feel what it is like to move, so he should get plenty of handling and changing of position in the pram or cot. Frequent changes of environment are good and he should have a variety of toys. Sometimes he should be put on the floor, but not always in the same place and on the same rug. In this way he gets to know the various textures of the furniture and surroundings and becomes adjusted to different temperatures.

Individual advice on these points is useful from the earliest stages. Physiotherapists like to meet and talk to the mothers and show them 'passive movements' especially suited to their baby, movements that are aimed at keeping the legs as strong as possible. They can also warn about certain mistakes such as, for instance, letting a toddler use a deformed foot too much. As well as paying heed to such warnings the parents of a spina bifida baby should encourage him to grow used to the floor as he soon learns to crawl about.

At about seven months the baby should be sitting. It is a good idea for him to have a special chair which will hold him upright and which has a large tray which surrounds him at almost shoulder level. Naturally the chair needs to be more or less indestructible so that other children can play at the tray without risk of breakage. The chair needs to be very firm so that it cannot be pushed over.

At this seven-month stage too the baby should be placed face downwards on the floor and encouraged to lift up his head and push up on his hands. Parents and physiotherapists can help at this period of his development by gently trying to compensate for the child's lack of free movement by seeing to it that as much movement as possible is retained by the joints. The physiotherapist can teach the parents to move the baby's toes up and down, to move his feet up and down, and to exercise the movement of his ankles. She can teach the parents special motions to help the knee and hip joints.

When the baby is about a year old, it is sometimes a good idea to use an adjustable 'crawler' of the type supplied by Zimmers Orthopaedics of 180 Brompton Road, London

S.W.3. This can be used until the child is about seven years old and is a popular means of exercise. Specially designed for its purpose this 'infant crawler' is strongly constructed of steel tubing and has a canvas sling covered with P.V.C. The child lies face down in the sling which takes his main body weight and uses his limbs to propel himself. The crawler is adjustable in height from eight to eleven inches. Another piece of apparatus that may be recommended for some children is the 'bonny bouncer', a sort of swing that can be hung in a doorway so that the baby can watch his mother doing her housework. This would help him keep abreast in development with a normal baby who would at this stage be crawling about after his mother and getting into everything.

Movements must be done slowly and with great care when the limits of the range of movement are reached, since the risk of fracture is always present. Whoever is exercising the child should make sure he has a full understanding of the aims of the treatment if this is to be carried out at home. Every step should be checked with the physiotherapist.

As he gets older the baby should be fitted with calipers and encouraged to stand with them. Occasionally a mother is not given clear enough instructions or perhaps does not take them in, and does not realise that the whole object is for the child to use the calipers to enable him to stand up, otherwise they are just dead weight for the child to drag around with him and they are worse than useless.

Here again the physiotherapist may be able to give treatment that will help the child prepare for calipers. She would probably teach him to establish equilibrium by alternating the pressure on his arms, showing him weight-bearing exercises and special ball games. She may be able to teach him to stand with a tripod and later to walk in parallel bars.

The next stage is to walk with tripods or crutches. Finally the child is taught to open doors himself. Being able to do this will be a very real part of his independence in life.

Spina bifida children are understandably afraid of falling but it has been found that they will happily play at trying to push the therapist over and fall with her! In fact at this stage the child pushes the therapist around quite a bit, but this encourages him to co-ordinate his movements and to learn to balance. The fear of falling is often particularly strong if the child has taken a long time to learn to stand alone. It is easier to teach a young child than an older one to lose his fear of falling, and this again shows why it is important for the spina bifida child to be taken as early as possible to the physiotherapist.

At home, any means of using and strengthening the child's arms and shoulders should be encouraged since his arms will have to carry not only his body weight but the weight of his calipers too. He should be urged to try to push himself up with his arms, to push against his parents, play ball games and other games involving the use of his arms, regularly and often. Some spina bifida children, for instance, thoroughly enjoy having wheelbarrow races with their playmates.

When a spina bifida child comes to the physiotherapy clinic with strong arms and shoulders, he can get around on crutches in a matter of months even if he did not start wearing calipers until he was six years old. However, as has already been stated, the spina bifida child should be put on his feet at the same time as an ordinary toddler would be.

These exercises at home do mean extra time to be given and perhaps further stress for the parents, who may feel they have just too much on their plate with the extra work they are already doing for their baby, and that this further task is one burden too many. This feeling is even more understandable if the calipers produce tears. However, calipers, it seems, never cause tears when they are put on at a clinic. Perhaps this is because there the children are given the idea that they put them on for their special play and activities, and of course there are other children around them doing the same thing.

In the clinic, once the calipers are on, the children are

always encouraged to stand. In some clinics about fifty children a day are put into calipers and then walk around happily. One child, a boy, was an example to everyone in his refusal to use a wheelchair as long as he could manage to walk. When his clinic group went on expeditions around the countryside a chair had to be taken for him, but the helpers were always pushing it around empty.

It goes without saying that calipers should always fit perfectly. Some children come to the clinic with calipers that are too big for them. Growth in the length and circumference of limbs causes a continually changing relationship between limbs and calipers. Growth is not always symmetrical and great care must be taken to see there is no undue pressure on the child's body in any area or at any point on the limbs. The calipers must be adjusted to fit in with the smallest changes in the child's body.

The children with the least degree of paralysis usually have small below-knee irons and these children, being more active than those with the longer, heavier ones, are liable to get more knocks and cuts and sore places if there is any rubbing by the calipers. Because his skin may be insensitive to pain the child may not feel any discomfort even if he has a sore, and so will not complain. This is something that has to be watched for constantly.

As mentioned in Chapter 3, it is important not to let the child put on too much weight. The lighter the handicapped child is the easier it will be for him to walk, and the less he will hurt himself when he falls over. Being light will help him too when he is learning to find his balance.

The normal child, in his early stages of walking, falls over and pulls himself up constantly. The only opportunity for learning to balance the spina bifida child has is when he is standing on his feet wearing his calipers. Since he has control only in the top half of his body he must learn to find his balance with that. All this exercising, training and preparation brings nearer the day when the child manages to take a few steps on his own.

The moments when the child first stands or first walks are cherished highlights in his life. It may be distressing for the unaccustomed onlooker to see a child struggling to walk with calipers and perhaps some other walking aids but to the child himself this movement is a thrill and a joy. It offers a whole new world of freedom to him and this independence represents a tremendous achievement on his part and is often the result of his own grit and the devotion and skill of the physiotherapist and the parents.

One child, on such an occasion, burst out with, 'This is the bestest day of my life. I've been waiting seven years for this!' He gazed happily at his reflection in the large mirror in front of him and, for the first time in his life, saw himself standing up. He was wearing calipers and holding on to parallel bars, but there he was, standing. He was nearer to behaving physically as his brothers and sisters did than he had ever been before.

In spite of the general pleasure and excitement that is felt by everyone concerned at such times, there should be no feeling of pressure or rush, as progress is likely to be slow for handicapped children. On the whole it is a matter of regular effort at the task of limb strengthening. A special table where the child can stand and play with his toys and where other children can join him is a great help in this. It has been found the children will stand playing for long periods, exercising and co-ordinating their muscles and enjoying themselves at the same time.

Care of the skin from the baby's earliest stages is another matter that is very important for the spina bifida child. On the other hand the child should not be 'wrapped in cotton wool', and toughening up the skin with soap, surgical spirit and talcum powder is recommended.

Because of sensory loss there is a risk that damage may be caused in many ways without the child being aware of it. For instance, all mothers have to be careful to see their children do not suffer from hot water bottle burns, nappy rash, pressure sores, and sores on the feet caused by unsuitable shoes. But the mother of the spina bifida child has to be doubly careful because if the sore place or wound is in the paralysed area, her child will not feel it and will not complain. This does not mean, unfortunately, that the sore will not become worse. It must be treated in good time and the source of trouble removed.

As the children grow older they should be taught to examine their skin regularly and often, and to be specially on the watch for sores after using new boots or appliances. They should keep a careful watch too on the trunk areas and the lower limbs. A specially angled mirror in the bathroom can help them do this.

Other dangers the children can be taught to look out for as they grow older are friction burns from rubbing calipers, burns from being too near sources of heat such as fires and radiators and having the bath water too hot. Then again sitting in one position for a long time can cause sores, and bedsores are a well-known hazard for the physically handicapped who tend to lie in one position. Foam mattresses and cushions can do much to help with the problems.

It is important to see the spina bifida child is warm enough, particularly keeping an eye on his paralysed limbs. If the limbs become blue and cold, the circulation can be improved by massage. The limbs should be stroked gently but firmly in an upward direction towards the heart. It is also helpful to raise the child's legs above the level of his heart for a few minutes several times a day. A pillow under his feet at night may also help the circulation.

Physiotherapists and parents have found there is much that can be done to help the child physically but it is important to remember to develop his character too. The disabled child should be allowed to take risks occasionally as other children do and any initiative he shows should be encouraged.

For instance if the children want to 'have a go' at various games they should be encouraged even if they seem unlikely to meet with much success. Like other people they must learn to take disappointments and to accept their limitations. It is important though to remember as well that a small success may be a great spur to further effort. Common sense all round is the ruling guide. Parents with doubts about any risks should consult the child's physiotherapist who will probably know the extent of his physical ability better than anyone else.

One of the greatest joys for handicapped people is to swim or splash about in a swimming pool. Exercises in warm water play a very real part in the therapy of nearly all spina bifida children. Apart from the benefit of the exercises there is the pleasure of floating and drifting, and perhaps swimming like 'ordinary' people.

For regular training in the swimming pool the therapist generally has about two children in the water. One child enjoys playing around holding on to the bar, while he waits his turn, the other child does his swimming movements either held up by his therapist or, when he can, on his own. Even some very badly brain-damaged children have shown a reaction of pleasure when introduced to water and have made efforts in that element they would never have attempted otherwise.

We sometimes forget that handicapped children are not a separate species. Their needs differ in degree rather than kind from those of other children. They may need extra help and special facilities and they certainly need more time spent on them, but the basic needs are the same.

If it seems daunting to read about all these recommendations that are given by the 'spina bifida families' and by the medical and welfare teams working with children with this handicap, it is perhaps worth recalling that if you wrote down the routine for a normal baby it would look fairly formidable, as many a father has discovered when taking over from his wife for a few hours! All babies and young children need practically round-the-clock surveillance, need tasks performed for them and like a lot of loving attention. In fact it is loving attention that the physiotherapists put first on their list as the spina bifida child's greatest need, speaking from their many years of experience.

If the parents can find the strength needed to train and help their child make the most of his abilities, if they can teach and encourage him in a matter-of-fact way, it will even be helpful to their own morale as well as being of great value to the child. There is so much the parents can do if they make the most of the baby's potentialities within the home during his waking hours, without depriving the rest of the family of love and attention.

Chapter 5

Help from the State

Much help is available for the handicapped in the United Kingdom. Most of the families I visited regularly took their children to hospital for check-ups and on the whole were aware of the various services available to them. However, conditions for the handicapped are gradually being improved so it is perhaps useful to indicate briefly what the overall situation is in this country.

All medical needs are generally met by the National Health Service, a service which includes the family doctor, hospital, maternity and other medical services. There are no prescription charges for children under fifteen. Certificates of exemption from prescription charges are available for people who suffer from certain conditions (these include a continuing physical disability which prevents them from leaving home except with someone else's help), for expectant mothers or a mother with a child under one year of age, for people who are getting supplementary benefit or family income supplement, and their dependants.

People not in any of these groups can still claim exemption or refund of charges if their income is not much above supplementary benefit level. For those who are not exempt and have to pay for frequent prescriptions, it is cheaper to buy a prepayment 'Season Ticket' certificate to cover all charges for six or twelve months. Leaflets giving information about prescription charge exemptions, refunds or prepayment certificates can be obtained from post offices or local social security offices.

Hospital services are free and do not depend upon the payment of any contribution. They include treatment as an in-patient, out-patient or day-patient. In-patient services include longer-term treatment and care of handicapped people who are in need of constant nursing attention. It is also sometimes possible for admissions to be arranged for short periods to give relief to relatives of handicapped people and the families of handicapped children.

For those who have to attend hospital either as an out-patient or day-patient, or who have children who have to attend and who cannot use public transport because of the disablement, or if there is no suitable public transport, special transport arrangements may be available. Again there is help here for those who are not well off. For those who are using public transport and are receiving supplementary benefit or family income supplement, fares to and from the hospital can be refunded on production of the order book or family income supplement exemption certificate when attending for treatment. People not receiving either of these benefits may still be entitled to help with fares if, because of low income, they are unable to meet the cost themselves. The hospital or local social security office can advise on how to claim.

Most families with spina bifida children are in touch regularly with the medical services but for those who are not and feel they are suffering from the strain of coping and would like the help of a social worker, contact should be made with the local authority social services department. Health visitors, for instance, make regular visits to see children at home and give advice to parents. They can also help in getting nursing aids and equipment. Then there are other free services that may be of use to the family with a spina bifida child or young person. For instance, some authorities supply incontinence pads, and some have a laundry service.

If the family live in a council flat or house and if in the local authority's view changes are necessary, the home can be adapted with the disability in mind. Local authorities can also help in the adaptation of private houses. Lavatory seats can be altered for instance, handrails can be provided, doors can be widened and sometimes an extra lavatory can be installed downstairs. Alterations and additions depend on what is needed and what is structurally possible The local housing departments have powers to give improvements grants in approved circumstances. To find out the position contact should be made with either the local health department or the local social services department.

Appliances such as crutches, calipers, walking aids and wheelchairs are supplied by the Department of Health and Social Security. Vandalism to public telephones which has rendered them useless, has sometimes brought prolonged discomfort to the handicapped child and anguish to the parents trying to contact their doctor or a hospital. Therefore in cases of real need, financial help for a home telephone may be available but not for the cost of the calls. For this concession the local social services department should be contacted.

Day nurseries or play groups provisions which can help care for handicapped children and do much to assist their development, are often provided. This kind of service may also be available during holidays for children who attend school. In some cases a charge may be made according to the family's means. For further information about this, contact should be made with the local social services department.

The local social services department may be able to help too in other ways. For instance, they may be able to offer advice and help with the problems that arise in bringing up and caring for a handicapped child. They work in close association with the medical and education services in trying to ensure that children and their families receive the support they need. This department can also help by contacting voluntary organisations which aim to bring together parents with the same family problems.

Many mothers looking after severely handicapped children are entitled to receive the attendance allowance. The attendance allowance is a tax-free cash benefit for people who are severely disabled physically or mentally, and who need a lot of looking after.

The medical requirements are, to use the words of the

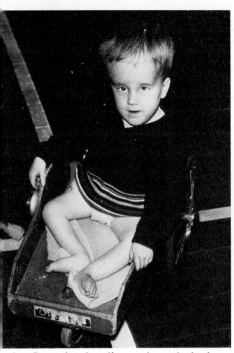

9. Severely handicapped and hydrocephalic child sitting in his trolley.

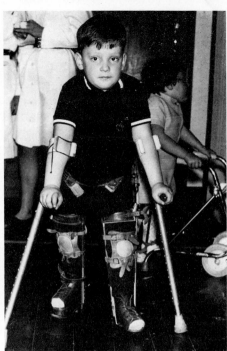

10. Keith, severely handicapped, with crutches and calipers.

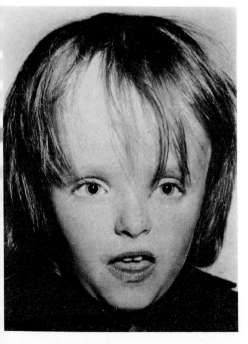

11. Elaine, hydrocephalic girl.

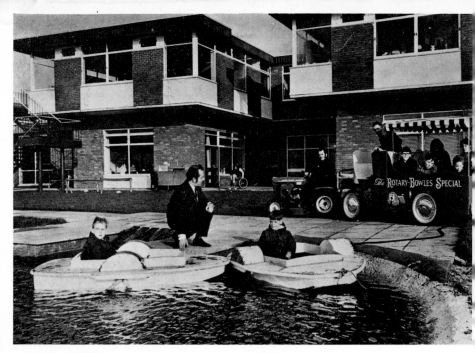

12. At a holiday home.

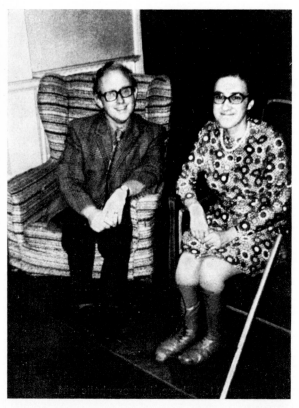

13. A married couple in their home. They both have spina bifida.

official leaflet, 'that a person must be so severely disabled physically or mentally that he requires frequent attention throughout the day in connection with his bodily functions, or continual supervision throughout the day in order to avoid substantial danger to himself or others and prolonged or repeated attention during the night in connection with his bodily functions, or continual supervision throughout the night in order to avoid substantial danger to himself or others'.

A child must satisfy the additional requirement that the attention or supervision required must be substantially in excess of that normally required by a child of the same age and sex. In the case of a disabled child, the allowance is normally paid to his mother, father or the person with whom he is living.

Where the conditions for attendance allowance are satisfied, the allowance for a child is paid to his mother if he is living with her. It may also be paid to the child's mother if the child is not living with her because he is in residential accommodation, provided that the mother and father are paying at least the amount of the allowance towards the cost of his accommodation. This does not apply if the residential accommodation is provided directly or indirectly by a local or other public authority. If the allowance is paid to the child's mother and she is a married woman living with her husband, the husband can draw the allowance but it belongs by law to the wife and it is she who must claim the allowance. 'Mother' includes step-mother and, in the case of a legally adopted child, the adoptive mother.

If the allowance cannot be paid to the child's mother, it may be paid to the father if the child is living with him – for example where the father is a widower. It may also be paid to the father if the child is in residential accommodation and the father is paying at least the amount of the allowance towards the cost of the accommodation. This does not apply if the residential accommodation is provided directly or indirectly by a local or other public authority. 'Father' includes step-father and, in the case of a legally adopted child, the adoptive father.

D

If the child is not living with the mother or father, the allowance may be paid to the person with whom the child is living. But if the mother or father or some other relative (i.e. a grandparent, brother, sister, step-brother, step-sister, half-brother, half-sister, and such a relative by adoption) is contributing towards the cost of providing for the child, it will be at the discretion of the Secretary of State to decide to whom the allowance should be paid.

Forms can be obtained from any local social security office who will also supply a stamped addressed envelope for the return of the completed form. A claim for a child should not be made before he is twenty-two months old. Attendance allowance cannot be paid for any period before the date of the claim. Once the claim has been made the Department will acknowledge it and will arrange for a medical examination to be carried out, usually by the disabled person's own doctor.

The Attendance Allowance Board or a doctor to whom they have delegated power decides whether a person satisfies the medical requirements. The Board is an independent body and is composed of medical practitioners and people from outside the medical profession, all of whom have a special interest and experience in the needs of the disabled. If the Board or one of their doctors decide that one or more of the medical requirements are satisfied they will issue a certificate and state a period during which one or more of the requirements have been, or are likely to be, satisfied.

If the Board or one of their doctors issues a certificate and all the other conditions are satisfied, attendance allowance will be awarded at the appropriate rate and the claimant will be notified in writing of the outcome of his claim. The notification will tell him of the courses open to him if he is dissatisfied.

Attendance allowance is normally paid by means of order books, and the orders can be cashed at a chosen Post Office. Whenever possible, payments to adults are combined with payments of other benefits, for example retirement or widows' pensions, invalidity benefit or supplementary benefit.

Attendance allowance is paid in full in addition to any national insurance benefits, industrial injuries benefits, or war pension.

Supplementary benefit is not affected unless it includes a special payment to meet attendance needs. In this case an adjustment will be made.

Payment of attendance allowance may be affected by:

The child's admission to hospital. (Other than as a 'private patient'.) Payment may continue for up to four weeks.

The child's admission to residential accommodation. This includes a 'home' of any kind or a school at which he stays overnight.

The child's absence from home on holiday or on a visit to relatives for more than four weeks. The allowance may then become payable to someone else.

The child's absence abroad.

The absence from home, for any reason, for more than four weeks of the person to whom attendance allowance is being paid for the child. The allowance might then become payable to someone else.

The reduction of payments towards the cost of providing for a child not living with the claimant.

Being with foster parents to whom a local authority is paying a boarding out allowance.

If attendance allowance is not being paid for a disabled child, because normally he is in hospital, in 'a home' or at boarding school, the allowance can be paid for periods when he is at home, for example on holiday or at weekends. Inquiries about payment should be made of the Department well before the disabled child is first expected to come home, particularly when no claim for attendance allowance has previously been made.

If a disabled child does not satisfy one of the special residence conditions above, the condition can be treated as satisfied if:

The claimant (usually the mother) satisfies the conditions appropriate to her, *or*

The claimant is a British subject whose place of birth is in the United Kingdom.

There are special conditions which help certain people to satisfy the residence conditions. These people are members of H.M. Forces; wives, children, parents and parents-in-law who accompany members of H.M. Forces abroad; members of the British Merchant Service; people going abroad for medical treatment; and nationals of certain countries with which there are reciprocal agreements on social security.

There are additional conditions which have to be satisfied by certain people such as members of foreign and Commonwealth forces stationed in the United Kingdom; representatives of overseas Governments; and certain officials of international organisations whose earnings or other emoluments are exempt from United Kingdom income tax, and their wives and children.

Special arrangements too exist to help certain people coming from another country which is a member of the European Economic Community to satisfy the residence conditions more quickly. Inquiries should be made at the local Social Security office if further information is needed about any of these special rules.

The many services provided to help people who are handicapped are described in a booklet *Help for Handicapped People* which is obtainable free from local social security offices and from the health and social services departments of local authorities. A copy is sent automatically to everyone who claims attendance allowance. For fuller details application should be made to the Department of Health and Social Security for leaflet N1205.

All local health authorities provide child health clinics staffed by doctors and health visitors who will give advice about the particular health needs of a child and about ways of encouraging his development.

If a child is being treated in a hospital which is some distance from home the parents may have difficulty in travelling to visit him, or in staying overnight near to the hospital, or in finding someone to look after other members of the family while they are away. Parents with this kind of problem should tell the hospital social worker and see if they can be helped in any way.

Parents worried about whether any future children born to them might be handicapped may arrange for genetic counselling at one of the Genetic Counselling Centres where the risk of a child being born handicapped can be calculated, as explained more fully in Chapter 7 of this book. The family doctor can arrange this counselling.

There are special educational facilities for handicapped children. These are dealt with in Chapter 6.

Chapter 6

Education and Training

The need for spina bifida children to have the best education from which they can benefit is particularly great because of their physical handicaps. This is not only the most reasonable and humane approach to the subject of education and training but it is also the most logical one for using the country's resources. People with spina bifida may never be able to take on a physically demanding job but they can use their abilities in all the other ways. With the exception of those who suffer from brain damage, they can use their minds for non-physical work or at least work demanding the minimal physical effort, and many light jobs are within their power.

The age we live in is, after all, the age of technology and more and more of the physical work is being done by machines. The able person in a wheelchair or walking with calipers can now achieve much through his ability to push the right button. With adequate education and training, people with this disability who have not suffered brain damage can become earners instead of being supported by their families or by the state. Jobs such as switchboard operating and many other office jobs may be suitable and certainly need not be dull or dead-end. Local authorities tend to be very helpful in assisting the disabled to find employment.

Educationalists consider it is better for the physically handicapped with normal intelligence to go to an ordinary school if possible and this is also what is wanted by most parents. On the whole both groups believe the child will get a wider education in an ordinary school and they believe too that he will benefit socially from it. However, ordinary schools are sometimes unable to take disabled children.

For those children for whom ordinary schools are not feasible there are special schools and these certainly offer some real advantages for the handicapped child. In some ways there is much less stress in these circumstances for the parents and the child. There is, for instance, freedom from worry that the child will run into difficulties through his incontinence or that he will fall short of the attainments of his fellows, or that things will, in some other way, go wrong since it is unlikely every other schoolchild will behave in an enlightened way towards his handicapped schoolfellow (although the incidence of teasing in ordinary schools seems to be extremely low).

These are some of the aspects to be taken into consideration when deciding what sort of school would be most suitable for the handicapped child. Others are the quality and sympathy of the teachers, transport facilities, the type of building and equipment, toilet facilities and the possibility of privacy, availability of helpers in the school in this connection, and availability of teaching aids. It is helpful too if the non-handicapped children have been prepared for the arrival of the handicapped child.

Many children who have spina bifida are able to attend an ordinary primary and secondary school and be accepted there, and enter into full school life without question, even to the point where, in some cases, the child's needs are overlooked or not realised. On the other hand, in some schools staff and pupils are so supportive that the handicapped child is given too much help. These, of course, are not the results looked for.

The staff concerned do need to know something about the difficulties of their pupils who have spina bifida and unfortunately in some cases they have received very little information and what they have received has come from the parents.

There is considerable overlap between the standards of physical handicap in ordinary and special schools. When making the choice between a normal and a special school the disadvantage of the stress of trying to manage in a normal school has to be balanced against the fact that the child will need to face up to normal people in the adult world. So far as educational standards are concerned, some special schools are able to carry out a near-normal school curriculum but the principal enemy they face, from the very nature of the selection of pupils, is loss of time when the pupils have check-ups and treatments. Medical and physical requirements have to take precedence over educational needs since a child who is ill cannot work properly. It is therefore difficult for the special schools to create a situation where the child is fully stretched intellectually. To allow for their lower stamina handicapped children attending special schools usually have shorter hours than the normal schoolday. It should be remembered too that it is not necessary to make a decision for all time in the matter of the type of school. The child may be able to start at a special school and then transfer to a normal one.

As with all children, the aim for the child with spina bifida is independence to the utmost extent possible, so that he or she may become a fulfilled, friendly young person, get the best out of schooldays, have a suitable training and finally take a job and lead an independent life.

The educationalists and physiotherapists I talked to all agreed that nursery school is of very special help to these children because, apart from the specific skills learned and tasks performed, the children become socialised, they become full citizens of their small world with all the checks and balances that young people use on each other. They learn, too, to be co-operative with the staff before they go to primary school.

I know from listening to parents that choice of school is sometimes difficult. The choice before them is between normal primary and secondary schools, special schools for physically handicapped children, special schools for educationally backward children, special schools for those who will not benefit from normal education, residential care homes, and hospital schools. Some very severely handicapped children may have to have home tuition.

There is great variation within the schools as so much depends on the staff and the area concerned. For instance, in many cases special arrangements may have to be made to deal with their incontinence if the children cannot attend to themselves or if they do not return home for lunch.

Changes of outlook and changes of problems are having their effects on all schools and particularly the special schools. Poliomyelitis and tuberculosis, for example, have virtually disappeared; the survival rate of children with spina bifida, by contrast, has gone up. Increasingly, therefore, efforts are being made to find ways of catering for the less severely handicapped children in primary and secondary schools.

The trend in the special schools in fact is to have more and more children with spina bifida and the intelligence level tends to decline. This is not so black a picture as it might seem since the reason for the drop in the level of mental ability is that more and more of the physically handicapped children with normal mental ability are being accepted in the ordinary schools. The reason for the rise in the number of children with spina bifida coming into the special schools is that more are surviving into school age and well beyond, and schooling can, in fact, offer them many benefits besides the obvious ones.

Intelligence tests often cause dissatisfaction among parents. Sometimes they see their child is alert, 'knowing', that he takes an active part in social conversation and yet he scores fairly low in the tests. It has been found that among spina bifida children in the 50:80 IQ range of intelligence, the parents commonly expect too much of them in tests.[1] Children with spina bifida tend to underscore in intelligence tests. At about eight years of age they score on average about twenty-five IQ points less than their siblings. One survey in this sphere found that in only two cases out of fifty did the spina bifida child score higher than his siblings.

[1] An 'intelligence quotient' of 100 represents the average intelligence level of the adult population of Great Britain.

Many parents are given an indication of what school would be suitable for their child as he approaches the age to go to primary school but for others, for instance for parents who have recently moved to a new area, the best course would be to go to the new education authority and ask for an assessment of their child. The needs of the child and the wishes of the family will be taken into consideration when a school is recommended.

The local primary school may or may not be suitable. If it is not, there will probably be a special day school in the area which will take in handicapped children and where the ratio of teachers and nurses to children is very high indeed. Then there is the possibility of a residential school where, in most cases, the children return home at weekends. These weekends at home are very important as they keep the family in contact with the child and the child does not feel abandoned.

The incontinence problem does not offer many difficulties in the early stages of education. In the nursery school the results of any accidents are cleaned up by an assistant and even in the infants' school teachers are used to the odd puddle. However, in the realms of secondary education, as stated earlier, special arrangements may have to be made for the incontinent child who cannot attend to himself. Unfortunately in some schools lavatories do not appear to be very private places, and missing locks may make life difficult for anyone who has to attend to himself in a way different from the rest of the pupils. Apart from aiming to keep washing and lavatory accommodation on as high a standard as possible, the problem remains one of coping with human curiosity and hoping that humanity and good manners prevail.

When choosing a school it is advisable to visit the head teachers in the area and to discuss the child's possibilities with them. On the whole, for cases on the borderline between normal and special schooling, it has been found better not to push matters too far when trying to get a child into an ordinary school. It is better for a child to go to a special school and then be transferred to a normal school because he has made so much progress, rather than the other way about. It is also better for the child to be fully accepted wherever he goes and not just tolerated. In some areas there are special units for handicapped children attached to normal schools.

Whatever school is selected, parents and school should make every effort to see these children are involved in every possible function. This attitude should continue during the holidays as well, and here the local parents' association may be of help.

Most readers are familiar with the normal schools of this country but perhaps a description of the facilities offered by some of the special schools should be given.

Special schools often offer excellent facilities. Preswylfa in Cardiff, South Wales, is a good example of a modern nursery school and assessment centre for children with multiple handicaps. It gives special early training. It is a light, modern school, on one floor with a pleasant feeling of openness built in a garden setting. The staff consists of a head teacher, three full-time teachers, three nursery nurses and a teachers' aid who helps mainly in the bathroom and with the meals.

The children are given special early training in bladder and bowel management and special treatment such as speech therapy and physiotherapy. Their age range is from two to seven years but they are mainly aged from three to six years. About one-third of them have spina bifida. The head-mistress talked about her school and about her spina bifida pupils with optimism and confidence.

'We've got a routine here and we've had some success,' she told me. 'I think there are great advantages for the child at a special school. For instance we have urine tests every fortnight to try to detect bladder infection early. We have our own therapist who helps the children with mobility and helps prevent further deformity.

'Then we act too as an advisory centre. If the mother is really stuck we are generally the first people who know about it. If we are in trouble we contact the paediatric health visitor.' Speaking of the mothers' participation in the school life, she said, 'Mothers can come into the school at any time but on the whole are not encouraged to come in to help regularly. The object is to give them a change. We have many volunteer workers though, especially at certain times such as during the school or college holidays.'

This school carries out continuous functional, medical and educational assessment of the children, if necessary, until the age of seven, pending a decision on the child's next school. Another advantage is that the school medical officer, who is also attached to the Department of Child Health in the Welsh National School of Medicine, visits weekly. Paediatricians too visit frequently. Besides these there are regular visits from the educational psychologist working in the special schools, and from the specialist health visitor. Special door-to-door transport is arranged and there is always an escort from the staff of the school, which means there is daily contact with the home. Further contact between parents and the school comes through the Parent/ Staff Association which is a thriving concern doing much to raise morale as well as funds which are put to good use.

When the child starts at this nursery school the mother usually comes as well for the first week so that she and the child can get to know the staff. Arrangements are made for the parents to meet the team dealing with their child at regular intervals. Even before enrolment the child is visited several times by the school medical officer and specialist health visitor, and a social and medical report is made on him. After admission and when the child has settled in it is possible to carry out more detailed examinations and find out more about his general intellectual level, and to give him some physical tests such as assessments of eyesight and hearing. Throughout his stay there a most careful watch is kept on him while he learns to play a part in life.

Chailey Heritage Craft School and Hospital is one of the most famous schools for very severely handicapped children. Technically this is a long-stay hospital for physically handicapped children. It has patients ranging from a few weeks to sixteen years of age. Of the 240 or so children there, about a hundred have spina bifida and their numbers are increasing yearly.

The school is situated in the beautiful countryside of Sussex and has a special atmosphere of which the staff are proud. In spite of the very severe physical defects of the children, miraculously, it is an atmosphere of school which predominates. A glance through a classroom window shows six or seven boys heading a football around, a visit to the classrooms may reveal an active class doing modern painting, or a group absorbed in woodwork. Only at second glance are you reminded by calipers, wheelchairs or some special apparatus, of the severe handicaps of the children. The whole emphasis is on the job or the game in hand. The

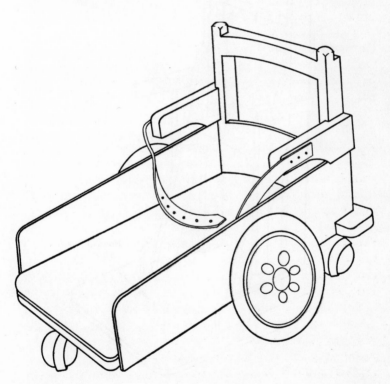

The Chailey Chariot.

class is a class of school children before it is a class of handicapped children.

This atmosphere of absorption with the job in hand is brought about by the dedication of the staff and the enlightened policy of the headmaster who puts education before vocational training or training for work. This means that the children's personalities stand a better chance of developing to their full potential and eventually they will

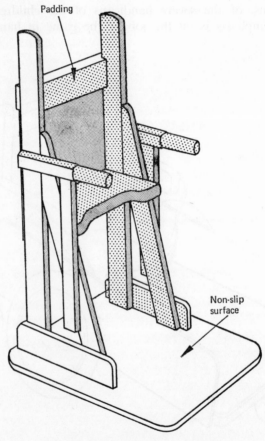

Padding

Non-slip surface

The Chailey Heritage Standing Chair.

take any training which may follow much more easily in their stride.

The children are first admitted for a trial period in the Admission/Assessment ward. After careful consideration of the physical, educational and social factors, a decision is made as to whether The Heritage seems the most suitable place for the child. Selection is based on the physical and intellectual disability and if it is decided it is in the child's best interests to remain he moves from the assessment ward to the ward or dormitory to which he has been allocated. The Heritage comprises an ambulant school, a hospital ward school and a resident medical block.

Decisions about a child's programme are discussed and made by a cross-section of the main professional staffs involved, and a considered plan is drawn up. In the case of the spina bifida child this combines a programme of bladder and bowel training, which includes the provision of special appliances such as urinals for the boys and, later, ileal loop equipment for the girls, to deal with incontinence. The bowel training programme is largely undertaken by the nursing staff. When the children arrive at the baby-toddler stage, the main aim is to get them moving independently. Out of this need evolved the Chailey Chariot which quite small children, aged about ten or eleven months, can use. The children then graduate to crutches with various other types of walking aids, usually including calipers with a trunk-support in the early stages which is then gradually reduced. This part of the mobilising programme is undertaken by the Physiotherapy Department. Certain problems of daily living independence for other aspects, including perhaps clothing modifications, are undertaken by the Occupational Therapy Department.

Most of the special equipment, such as standing-tables and modified chairs, are designed and made in the Experimental Workshop, as are quite a variety of other aids for disabilities. Experimental work is going on in a number of directions in the Workshop. One project, for example, is a lighter type of caliper. They are also trying to improve other sections of equipment.

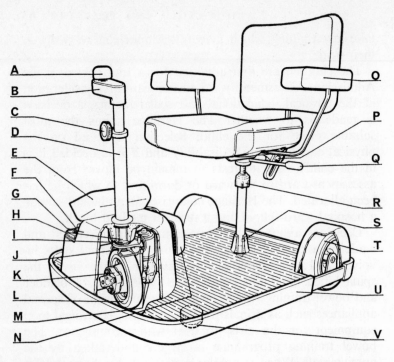

A	Control knob	I	Thrust needle bearing	P	Chair back adjustment
B	Control box and steering tiller	J	Power contact points	Q	Seat locking lever
C	Column height adjustment knob	K	Cushion drive Coupling	R	Seat height adjustment
D	Control column	L	Drive and steer wheel	S	Grub screw for chair removal
E	Battery lid			T	Rear wheels
F	Battery	M	Drive motor and gear box	U	Buffer strip
G	Battery and power unit housing	N	Battery charger (in charging position)	V	Anti-tip pads
H	Control column socket	O	Leabank chair with moveable arm rests		

A chair that might be useful for adults is the 'Chairmobile'. It was invented by Lord Snowdon for his friend, Quentin Crewe, who is a disabled journalist. Easy to drive and steer, it is meant for indoors, is smaller and more easily manœuvred than a wheelchair. It is powered by a rechargable battery and travels at 0·7 miles per hour. The *Sunday Mirror* has arranged to sell the first 2,500 Chairmobiles at a price of about £100.

The orthotist (he used to be known as the appliance-maker), who works under contract, does the main supplying of the basic caliper equipment. He also supplies a new type of standing/moving supports known as 'parapodia'.

From these points it can be seen that the programme is essentially one of well-integrated teamwork and this is achieved through regular case conferences on the children when progress is regularly reviewed, and any modifications in the programme can be agreed between the appropriate sections of staff.

Psychological assessment of the child's potential obviously plays an important part in working out a satisfactory programme and for this the Senior Psychologist is a key member of the team. This assessment is a guide from the educational point of view for the teaching staff and also a lead to what one can expect, in progress with the therapy staff, whether this be the Physiotherapist, the Occupational Therapist or the Speech Therapist.

When the children are older, they do exercises that build up the arm, shoulder and trunk musculature. They learn to speed up their movements and this helps the children to move around more rapidly in everyday life. They perform these exercises in classwork with the Senior Remedial Gymnast.

Clearly, there are many background problems over such matters as housing, access to homes, need for ramps, and modifications in baths and lavatories. All of these are gone into by the Senior Medical Social Worker and, where necessary, supporting medical certificates are supplied to back the need for home modifications, where clearly these could make a great deal of difference to the burden on the parents.

Orthopaedic surgery that may be required is carried out by a visiting Orthopaedic Consultant, except in one or two cases of very major surgery of a specialised type, such as surgery for the spine, which is done at a special unit in London, at the Royal National Orthopaedic Hospital.

Another feature of The Heritage is the provision of day-rooms attached to the hospital wards. These enable the

E

children to get away from the bed area for the main part of the day, an arrangement which provides a more satisfactory pattern from the ward teachers' point of view. There is the further advantage that it provides more ample space for recreational activities, such as films and live shows.

Originally founded for seven boys from the East End of London, the school is now co-educational, although boys and girls are separated in the wards. In the early days the school concentrated on vocational training such as shoemaking, silversmith work and sewing. Nowadays they aim at giving the children a good education and encouraging business studies. The headmaster believes in streaming since it is impossible to teach children of wide intelligence range at the same time. He believes too that no craft training should be done at the expense of general education, and that there should be no craft training at all until the age of sixteen. On the other hand a large part of the staff's work is preparing the children for leisure unless, of course, the children happen to be compulsive readers, when this is less necessary.

Gardening is part of the children's education for leisure. They have a large greenhouse at The Heritage and every child can do almost everything aided by some of their special tools. There is a strong community sense among the children. The Chailey Heritage Old Scholars' Association is more than 600 strong.

The most modern teaching methods are used. Machines are used for the teaching of mathematics – one machine per child. Electric typewriters are used and so are tape-recorders. There is special school equipment for the hospital ward and even woodwork can be done in bed if necessary because there is a specially constructed workbench. There is a small electric car skilfully managed by one little girl who would be quite unable to get about without it. The classrooms have standing chairs and adjustable tables. In this hospital school for the severely handicapped the main problems, in fact, of the child who has spina bifida are not so very great. The teachers speak with some experience since almost all the intake nowadays is of children who have spina bifida.

The hospital is run by a team of four doctors and 340 staff of all disciplines, many of whom are part-time. Many organisations help and there are about sixty voluntary workers at the three sites of the hospital. They are lucky in benefiting from an enormous amount of goodwill from the local community. The hospital is visited regularly by consultants and by doctors from all over the world.

At the age of fourteen the children are carefully assessed, taking into account their educational ability, their physical ability and so on. They may then be given guidance as to the types of employment that come within their competence. They may stay at the hospital until they are seventeen. Then comes 'the moment of truth' since many of the pupils have by then been in the hospital for thirteen years. Some of them will find work, probably helped by the career officer, and others will go to have vocational training for periods of from one to three years. The highest proportion will go into sheltered workshops. A few students get into universities but most of them are educated up to 'O' level standard in various subjects.

Some of the children who live nearby have their weekends at home. Chailey Heritage has the ordinary three school terms and the ambulant children can go home for their holidays.

The strong emphasis on education, training for personal independence, and the development of character, the high morale, the excellent equipment available, make the onlooker feel that the child who comes here is indeed lucky. In spite of all they can do, however, the staff are aware of many social problems such as some of the children being rejected by their parents and needing substitutes, and the need for strong support for parents of all kinds.

Residential schools vary in their systems but most have ordinary school holidays. Parents are encouraged to visit and telephone their children and often the children go home every weekend to keep home ties as close as possible. Sometimes older pupils choose to stay for the weekends in their school to watch a football match or some similar activity. This element of choice also gives them a measure of independence. Most of the special schools will keep the children on until they are seventeen years of age if they can still benefit from the facilities given.

The official position of handicapped children in this country is laid down in the Education (Handicapped Children) Act which became effective in 1971. The law finally became truly all-embracing then in that the mentally handicapped were included, one hundred years after the Education Act, 1870. As stated in Chapter 1, some children with spina bifida have suffered brain damage. Reports on education from the Department of Education and Science explain the advantages of the Act for the mentally handicapped. The educational needs of children in training centres, in hospitals for the mentally handicapped, in independent special care units for children with serious physical disabilities or behaviour disorders, in private institutions or being cared for at home are to be considered along with those of children already in special schools. They are no longer classified as 'ineducable'.

It is now recognised that children who are severely handicapped mentally and physically have the same basic requirements as non-handicapped children. They need affection, security and a range of experiences through which their minds and bodies can develop, they too need opportunities to succeed and gain praise.

Nowadays many of the practices typical in normal nursery and infant education are gradually being included in the programmes of training centres and hospitals. Classrooms now offer a variety of learning situations to meet individual needs of children who learn less readily than normal children. Emphasis is placed on learning from real life and on social training. Even a little progress can make an enormous difference to the quality of their lives.

In recent years there has been rapidly growing interest in developing the potentials of mentally handicapped children and considerable material progress has been made. For instance new training centres have been provided, some with well-equipped nurseries, home craft units, workshops and swimming pools.

Another achievement has been the development of a system of training for teachers of the mentally handicapped. The academic qualifications of students on these courses have been steadily rising and those successful in qualifying have usually shown a strong sense of vocation and a high level of professional competence.

With regard to the education of the physically handicapped, Local Authority educational establishments are required by the Chronically Sick and Disabled Persons Act 1970 to make provision, so far as is practicable and reasonable, for the needs of disabled persons using the buildings, making sure access with walking aids or wheelchairs is possible and that parking facilities and suitable sanitary conveniences are available.

It is recognised too that physical education can be of great benefit to the physically handicapped. Swimming, canoeing, fishing, archery and camping are among some of the activities enjoyed by physically handicapped children today. An illustrated pamphlet *Physical Education for the Physically Handicapped* (HMSO), published by the Department of Education and Science describes the range of activities being undertaken in the special schools for the physically handicapped. The booklet urges schools to provide some of the various types of physical activities described and asks them to experiment further and to encourage physically handicapped young people to enjoy the satisfaction and fun that result from taking part in physical activity or recreation.

Parents often wonder how their handicapped child will manage at the end of his school days. The lightly handicapped will probably be able to fit in with the able-bodied but for the more severely handicapped, assessment and training facilities are available at residential colleges for the disabled and at government training centres.

There are also residential training colleges sponsored by voluntary organisations which offer a variety of technical, clerical and practical courses for men and women from the age of sixteen upwards, with a view to preparing them for employment in open industry. At St Loye's College,

Exeter there is a Further Education Unit which includes a functional assessment unit.[1]

Sheltered workshops and welfare workshops cater for a wide variety of disabilities and provide training for many different types of practical work. Great care should be taken to see that the handicapped school-leaver is sent to training that is suitable for him and will lead him to the correct level of employment. This means he should not necessarily take the first vacancy arising but should wait for the one appropriate to his ability so that his work will be not just a means of livelihood, but also a source of interest and satisfaction.

Adult education, training and employment do not, strictly speaking, come within the scope of this book but some data is given here so that parents and children may have an idea of what the possibilities are.

The Scottish Branch of the British Red Cross, for example, run two establishments for the care and training of the young adult disabled, one at Inverness, and one at Largs. The aim of these units is to develop the full health potential of the severely physically handicapped of both sexes between the ages of sixteen and thirty-five and, having done so, to maintain this level for as long as possible.

The individual's development possibilities are looked at with four aspects in mind: his private and personal potential, his social potential, his cultural and recreational potential and his occupational activity potential. The screening, assessment and supervision of progress and the rehabilitation programmes are under the direction of a highly qualified and experienced panel. Other residential establishments have work centres and sheltered workshops for the disabled but those run by the Red Cross in Scotland are particularly interesting in that they have three stages of work progression through which members learn and develop at their own rate. They are probably also unique in their 'positive health'

[1] For those looking for employment and advice, help should be sought from the careers officer of the Youth Employment Office. Some local authorities have special officers who have received additional training to guide the handicapped.

approach which, although less tangible in its advantages, is also of vital importance.

The first stage in this scheme is an occupational centre in which simple tasks of work are performed which may, incidentally, be specifically therapeutic. The second stage takes place in the work centre where there is a longer working day and more emphasis is put on the quality and quantity of work turned out. In both these stages the work is mainly of the light assembly type and is provided by the sheltered workshop, which is the third stage. Here, the employees (as they are by now) put in a full working day, paying income tax, national insurance and so on. Some employees progress from this stage to open employment or go to another sheltered workshop in their home area. Some residents, however, are not able to progress beyond the first and second stages.

The scheme is planned on an industrial assembly basis. In addition there is a new development at Red Cross House, Largs, which will enable residents, particularly those who may be leaving to marry or live in the community, to cook, do housework, budget, and run a home. This will be in addition to the other work, and both men and women will be able to participate.

The centre at Largs consists of The House, The Hostel, the three Occupational Activity Units, the gymnasium, and The Social and Home Training Unit in the specially adapted Lodge House. The House provides homely living conditions for most of the newly admitted residents and those attending the occupational and work centres. There is dormitory accommodation for male residents and there are mainly single rooms for the female residents. There are also a lounge, dining room, games room and a quiet room. The Hostel provides residential accommodation for those who are employed in the Sheltered Workshop. There is a greater degree of independence here than in The House.

Efforts are made to create conditions similar to those in the community at large. The Occupational Activity and Work Units consist of the Occupational Centre, the Work Centre and the Sheltered Workshop. At Largs, these units, although within the same grounds, are quite separate from The House and The Hostel, so that the residents have a separate place for work and home. Everyone is encouraged to make use of the social and recreational facilities available in the surrounding community.

At Inverness, the Red Cross House is purpose-built and incorporates the Occupational Therapy and the Work Centres. The Workshop is situated in a factory building on the local industrial estate, a mile or two from Red Cross House. The employees travel by car or by public transport. This workshop is open too to commuters from Inverness and the surrounding district, and so is the one at Largs.

The parent workshop, Haven Products Limited, Glasgow, is not residential but draws disabled employees from all over Glasgow and the surrounding area, employees being drawn from the ordinary working age group. A few of the residents from Largs and Inverness may eventually work there, living in lodgings, hostels or travelling from home.

These Red Cross establishments cater for adults suffering from spina bifida and other handicaps. They do not provide accommodation for married couples. However, the Thistle Foundation in Edinburgh can do this although in general they prefer one of the partners to be ambulant. When two residents from Red Cross House, Largs, were married, one of whom had spina bifida, they were able to move in there.

Chapter 7

Genetic Counselling

Any couple who are considering starting a family, but who are worried in case they should bring a handicapped baby into the world, should seek genetic counselling. It is far easier to put up with the disappointment of realising it would be unwise to risk starting a pregnancy and to plan life accordingly than to suffer the unhappiness of giving birth to a severely deformed baby.

What happens in a genetic counselling consultation? The counsellor interviews husband and wife together. At the beginning of the interview he tries to discover why the couple have come to him for advice, what they wanted from the interview and what the real problem is since this may not be exactly the one expressed by the couple. It might happen, for instance, that one of the couple, let us say the wife, feels she cannot probe too deeply into her husband's family history in the sensitive matter of congenital abnormalities. She knows, however, that the counsellor can do this with the minimum amount of offence. The counsellor asks what kind of birth control, if any, the couple have been using, whether the wife had any miscarriages and so on. Other important factors in this connection are the mother's age, the father's occupation and the location of the home.

The counsellor would ask questions about the couple's respective families. He would want as complete a picture as possible of the family tree of the husband and wife, going back at least one generation and more if possible and, in fact, gleaning any information he could of any abnormalities that may have occurred. It is a good idea for the couple to find out as much as possible beforehand from all their relatives. Such inquiries sometimes produce some hitherto unknown facts, since sad events such as babies dying and still-births are often considered, from the best possible motives, 'best forgotten'. However, for the purposes of genetic consultations all such information should be revealed.

When the counsellor thinks he has drawn out all the appropriate information available he calculates the couple's chances of having an abnormal child in the light of their entire background. The prospective parents should make the decision whether to try to have a baby or not, and the counsellor should not push them one way or the other. The various possibilities and risks are simply put before the clients.

Take the imaginary case of Mr and Mrs Brown. Mrs Brown had been 'on the pill' for two years after having given birth to a stillborn spina bifida child. Mrs Brown decided that before trying to become pregnant again, and perhaps risking giving birth to another malformed baby, she would seek advice.

Replying to the counselling doctor's questions, she said she was eldest of four, that she had a sister who had had an anencephalic baby, a brother with four normal children and a brother of seventeen who was not married. She knew her mother had had two stillborn babies before she had been born but it had always been assumed that these had been normal babies. Her mother had never discussed the matter with her family before her death and there was no one alive who could give them any reliable facts. Mrs Brown's uncle and aunts were normal and so were their children, two in each case.

Mr Brown was the second of eight children and there was no evidence of any abnormality in any of them or in their children, or in Mr Brown's parents or uncles or aunts.

Spina bifida and other malformations of the neural system are taken together when making calculations for genetic purposes. Mr and Mrs Brown were told the risk of their having a child with any of these conditions was about one in fifty and the risk of having a spina bifida baby was one in a hundred. The 'population' risk when there is no occurrence in the family is about one in 150 and one in 300 respectively. However the sort of risks the Browns would run can be very greatly reduced nowadays by making use of diagnostic facilities which can detect anencephaly and most forms of spina bifida in the first half of pregnancy which is early enough for an abortion to be carried out if indicated.

Having heard what the chance of bringing a handicapped child into the world would be, the couple may decide to accept the risk and encourage pregnancy, making use of the diagnostic facilities available. They may decide to postpone a decision until later when ante-natal diagnostic facilities may be more certain. On the other hand they may find the risk too high especially if they could not accept the possibility of an abortion. A couple who already had normal children might well decide not to take a risk. They might decide instead to try and adopt a child and perhaps follow this decision with contraceptive measures, or one of the couple might have an operation for sterilisation.

It helps to get matters into perspective if one considers that in any pregnancy there is a one in thirty risk of a child being born with any of the many known abnormalities, and the additional risk run because there is some spina bifida in the family is really quite small.

The prospect of bearing a spina bifida baby then is clearly more worrying than that of bearing an anencephalic one since in cases of anencephaly not only is the child stillborn but the condition can be detected in early pregnancies by a simple test which carries no appreciable risk. Most cases of spina bifida can now also be detected but this involves a procedure at about four months after conception which may have some small risk of causing an abortion.

Any couple who wish may have professional genetic guidance but the following hypothetical cases will show some of the problems that prompt couples to seek help. Mr and Mrs Blake, for example, had been married ten years and during that time Mrs Blake had had two miscarriages and, last year, had given birth to an anencephalic baby who had died at birth. This couple wanted to know where they stood with regard to starting a family so they arranged to have genetic counselling.

Assessing their family background, the counsellor learnt that Mrs Blake was twenty-eight years old, Mr Blake was thirty-two. Mrs Blake had been an only child but Mr Blake had a sister with a spina bifida occulta who had had no handicap to speak of. He had also had a baby brother who had been anencephalic and had died soon after birth.

The counsellor calculated that their risk of having a baby with an abnormality of the central nervous system was at least one in fifteen and their chance of having a baby with spina bifida was about one in twenty-five.

The Hawkins decided to seek genetic counselling as they had married rather late in life and they had heard that spina bifida babies were more likely to occur when the mother is in one of the extremes of the child-bearing group, either the older or the very young group. Mrs Hawkins was thirty-five years of age and Mr Hawkins was forty. Mrs Hawkins was one of a family of four and had three brothers. There had been no congenital abnormality in her family as far as she knew. Her husband had been an only child and there had also been no known congenital abnormality in his family. The counsellor assessed that the chance of their baby having one of the central nervous system abnormalities was less than one in 150, and the chance of their baby having spina bifida was one in 300. This, of course, is the 'population' risk, i.e. the risk that any pregnancy runs of resulting in one of these malformations.

The Mackenzies brought their problem to the counsellor. Mrs Mackenzie, aged thirty, had been married before and had had two children by her former husband, one of whom, the older one, a boy, had had spina bifida cystica. The second child, also a boy, was quite normal. In this case the geneticist needed to know the background of both husbands as far as possible in order to determine the risks for this couple and a second interview had to be arranged as Mrs Mackenzie had not realised that information about her former husband would be needed. The former husband and his family were co-operative when they were told the reason for the inquiries.

Mrs Mackenzie's first husband had been one of three normal children and his parents, uncles and aunts had also been normal. He too had married again but had had no children. Mrs Mackenzie's present husband, aged thirty-five, was an only child whose parents, uncles and aunts had all been normal. So far as he knew there was no congenital abnormality of any kind in his family. Mrs Mackenzie herself had no abnormality nor had her only sibling, a brother. Her father had been perfectly normal but her mother had always complained about pain in her back and had had 'something wrong'. She had died when Mrs Mackenzie had been quite young and her father too was now dead. It was thought by other members of the family that Mrs Mackenzie's mother had had some small back deformation.

Having had a spina bifida child (now aged five), Mrs Mackenzie knew how much extra work and stress was involved but she was still prepared to take a reasonable risk. She asked the geneticist whether an even longer wait after her first spina bifida baby would improve her chances of having a normal baby. These were the results of the geneticist's calculations. The risk of Mrs Mackenzie having another spina bifida baby was less than one in thirty. The length of the gap between the birth of the babies is not thought to affect the risk of recurrence.

Mrs Davies sought genetic counselling before starting a family since she herself had spina bifida occulta. She had suffered no hardship from this but wanted to know whether she was likely to give birth to a baby who might have a more severe version of her own malformation. Mrs Davies is twenty-two, one of six children. She was the only one with a congenital malformation. Her mother and father, aunts and uncles were all perfectly normal in this respect. Mr Davies is twenty-three. He is normal and so were his brother, his parents, aunts and uncles. The geneticist thought that the risk was probably no more than the 'population' risk (i.e. one in 300 for central nervous system malformations) as the spina bifida occulta in Mrs Davies' case was thought to be of no significance.

Children and young people with spina bifida may wonder what risks lie ahead for them when they become adults, marry and are thinking of having children. With so many more people with spina bifida reaching adulthood inquiries are coming from couples where one or other or both have one of the forms of spina bifida.

Their risk of having a spina bifida baby where only one of the couple has spina bifida seems to be as high as in the case of Mr and Mrs Brown – that is the risk of having a child with any of these conditions was about one in fifty and the risk of having a spina bifida baby was one in a hundred.

However, all these cases are only given as examples as each family is a problem on its own and numerous other factors have to be taken into consideration before coming to a decision in each particular case.

A lot of couples seek genetic counselling because a close relative such as the mother, an aunt or a sister has given birth to a spina bifida baby. In these circumstances the risk is very much less than if the couples themselves had had one. Genetic counselling should always include advice on contraception and family planning. Medical centres and social workers can assist couples in getting advice and practical help in preventing conception and in arranging for genetic counselling interviews for those who want them.

Chapter 8

Holidays

Everyone needs a holiday sometimes, particularly parents. If one of their children is handicapped the need of the parents for a change of surroundings and a break from duties is even greater. The Cardiff team of medical specialists working with spina bifida children and their families felt this very strongly. They realised that because of the extra burdens they bore, all such families should be given an opportunity of rest from immediate worries by having a holiday with or without the spina bifida child.

Many factors operate when parents are taking the difficult decision whether to take their holiday with or apart from their disabled child. They feel torn between the desire to keep the child with them and the awareness of their own need for rest. Other factors they have to consider are what facilities are available, how the other members of the family would be affected and, most important, how the disabled child would feel.

It is a surprise to some parents to find that many children who go away separately enjoy themselves and derive positive benefit from being away from the family for a short time. A separate holiday can give the handicapped child a feeling of independence, particularly as he grows older. He sees the world from a different angle and can have plenty to tell the family when he returns home. It also helps to prepare the child to face such breaks with the family as may come later because of schooling or training or some other reason.

In an ideal community holidays for all families would be taken for granted. Even in the imperfect world of today certain facilities such as holiday homes, chalets and caravans

have been made available by ASBAH (the Association for
Spina Bifida and Hydrocephalus), and other societies, to
help those with disabled children.

For instance, near Cowbridge in South Wales there is the
Jane Hodge Holiday Home built on a seven-and-a-half acre
site. This Home serves the physically handicapped children
of Wales and the Border Counties and has guests with a
wide range of handicaps such as cerebral palsy, muscular
dystrophy and thalidomide damage, as well as spina bifida.
A stay here, as many of the children will tell one is a
great annual treat. The place seems like paradise to the
youngsters as so much that is beyond their scope normally
is here brought within their grasp. Besides this they make
friends and contacts who enrich their lives. This Home, for
example, was lucky enough to be adopted by a naval ship.
The ship's company invited the children on board for a
party, allocating two sailors to every child. As can be
imagined everyone had a rollicking time and the children
talked about it for days. Some made pen-friends among the
sailors.

The Jane Hodge Home has a hydrotherapy pool where
the children splash around, float and swim. There is a
super-aquatic roundabout on which even the most disabled
can be put into chairs, swung into the centre of the pool and
whirled round in the water. In this kind of element many of
the physically disabled lose their feeling of handicap. They
can relax and enjoy a new freedom. No parents, however
active and devoted, can keep up the momentum a team of
willing and skilled workers can achieve.

True to the holiday spirit of the Home, the aim in the
swimming pool is to have thrills, fun and enjoyment rather
than therapy; this is an important part of the annual twelve-
day treat. Everything is designed to make life as easy as
possible both for the children and for those looking after
them. There are always two able-bodied supervisors in the
water and one on the side. There are hooks at the side of the
pool for the wheelchairs.

In this little world the house father is at the centre of the
fun. Besides watching over the children, teaching them and

helping them, he creates 'disturbances' by hitting the water with tremendous smacks. The splashes bring squeals of delight from the young bathers and the scene is watched with smiles and chuckles by the two or three children at the side who have not gone into the water. The echoing sounds of happiness coming from the pool are as whole-hearted and boisterous as any parent could desire.

To deal with incontinence, the children are toileted before going into the pool and those who need it wear special protection. The water is kept at between 85 and 90 degrees winter and summer. It is tested daily and the plant is self-chlorinating and self-filtering. Children use a handrail to get into the pool or slide into it on their bottoms, loudly encouraged by those already in.

Sometimes older age-groups come to this home. One young man had his eighteenth birthday party there and invited some of his able-bodied friends to see what he could do in the water. It is hard to think of an instance that would demonstrate more clearly the pride the disabled person feels when he finds in the water the power to move about on his own that is denied him on dry land.

Every room in this Home has a holiday atmosphere and has something to add to the children's interest. There is a play-room, a music-room which has the added attractions of a television set, and a bird-cage full of live budgerigars. There is a grotto with gnomes, and everywhere you look there are dolls and large cuddly teddy bears.

The bedrooms are light and airy with large windows overlooking the hilly countryside. There are specially built bathrooms and lavatories in the dormitories, a toy on every bed, and an 'early to bed' room to ensure enough sleep for those who need more than the others. Altogether the place manages to combine modernity with homeliness in a marvellous way.

Outside the building there is a whole world of adventure for the children. There is a boating lake with special safety-paddle boats. A sturdy rocking 'boat' stands in the playground. Then there are log cabins, a pets' corner, an adventure playground, a crazy golf course, swings, a 'surrey with the fringe on top' in which the children go for rides, drawn by their own tractor, and there is an old van painted in psychedelic colours. All toys around the place have been given by well wishers and it is heartening to see what voluntary aid can achieve. Indeed the Home itself is testimony to that.

The young holiday-makers here do not remain within the walls of the Home. They get about and are a familiar sight being driven round the countryside in their own bus which has an electric hoist for the wheelchairs, and is also specially equipped inside. Their picnics and outings generally include a stop at one or two shops where the owners do not mind the long and deep consideration needed over what gifts the children will take home to their families.

A large skilled and devoted staff is required, for all this, as can be imagined. It is essential that there should be nursing staff with full SRN qualifications, house mothers and house fathers with experience in child care and entertainment, experienced cooks and kitchen staff providing tasty and well-balanced meals, domestic staff to ensure the highest possible standard of hygiene, maintenance staff to service the centre, with its special equipment and grounds, and administrative staff.

Capable volunteer workers are also an important part of the organisation and help of this kind is given generously. For instance the RAF and the Police supply drivers for the special day trips. Great interest is shown locally on all open days and young people from Atlantic College, a sixth-form school not very far away, regularly work there as volunteers.

This Home has been described fairly fully to give some idea of how much it and others like it may have to offer the disabled child. When parents know their child can enjoy such a holiday it gives the rest of the family the chance to travel and relax in a more carefree way than is usually possible for them when one of the members is disabled. The family can go away with peace of mind, knowing that their child is in good hands, looked after by qualified staff and devoted volunteers, in a specially designed building.

In cases where the parents are planning a separate holiday

but a holiday home scheme is not feasible, it is possible to arrange for the handicapped child to be cared for in a hospital-school or hospital. The local authorities, the family doctor or the health visitor are the people to give help in making such arrangements.

Ten-day Junior Red Cross holidays, run by the British Red Cross during the summer, are another possibility. These holidays are organised in carefully selected buildings and are run by someone experienced in dealing with children, such as a teacher, and there is a trained nurse in attendance. There also has to be access to a local doctor who is told in advance about the children's various handicaps. The handicapped children are generally the guests of the Society and are looked after throughout the holiday by members of the Junior Red Cross.

Every child applying to go to one of these holidays is visited beforehand by either an experienced Red Cross Officer or a local authority welfare officer who can assess the child's disability and needs, and talk to the parents and the child about the holiday. It has been found that visits beforehand and a talk about the holiday help prevent homesickness, and ensure that the children know someone when they arrive at the holiday centre. The assessment of the child's needs is most important. Incontinence is no bar but the organisers must know how much help will be needed. They will use their discretion to decide whether their holiday home is suitable for that particular applicant. These holidays are not suitable for the mentally handicapped.

Holidays for handicapped children play an increasing part in the British Junior Red Cross Society's programme. They start planning nine months beforehand to try to make the holiday as carefree and adventurous as is possible for their particular group of charges.

During the holiday the emphasis is on maximum participation, and the children enjoy games, singing at the camp-fire, and working with their own group of Junior Red Cross Cadets and other handicapped children. The Red Cross believe in taking children with a variety of handicaps as they find the campers can help each other so much. They are in the open air as much as possible and a camp-like atmosphere is strongly encouraged. Transport to and from the holiday centre is often arranged by voluntary bodies.

The Red Cross like to remain in contact with the young visitor after he has returned home, particularly if he is not getting much young companionship. Several branches of this organisation have formed special clubs for handicapped children and meet weekly, fortnightly or monthly during the year, and there the happy companionship between guests and Cadets formed during the holiday can be maintained.

These are just some of the possibilities that exist for giving the handicapped child and his family separate holidays. There are other homes throughout the country dealing with the full range of handicaps.

In cases where the disabled child is going with the rest of the family, there are specially adapted caravans or chalets in the holiday areas of England and Wales that may be rented or, in some cases, lent free. In fact, families who cannot afford the rental stay rent-free and are given some spending money, and in many instances private volunteers will drive them to their destination and collect them. Families wanting to know what is available for them should make inquiries through their local branch of ASBAH. There are other organisations too that are anxious to give help to the families where one of the members is handicapped.

Sometimes the greater the need for the holiday, the harder it is to arrange because of all the complications involved. Then too the tireder the parents are, the less energy they have to make any extra arrangements. One mother I interviewed had not had a holiday for twelve years. By this time she did not feel any real urge for one but surely no one could doubt the very great need for it.

Another mother I interviewed had thoroughly enjoyed her holiday with her husband and her two children in the special 'spina bifida' caravan in Porthcawl. Their little boy who had spina bifida had by chance met a little spina bifida girl. Seeing his back when he wore his bathing trunks she said to him, 'That's good. You've had the same operation as me!'

Grandparents frequently play an important role at holiday time, helping to share the work and, perhaps more important, the child-minding, so giving the parents a chance to have some hours on their own. In fact, never have all the mother-in-law jokes seemed so hopelessly misplaced as in the situation of a couple having a handicapped child where Granny and Grandpa often act as the most loving and helpful substitute parents.

Chapter 9

The Possibilities of Independence

What the future holds for their children is naturally one of the questions most troubling to parents. I found that when this subject arose in interviews parents were extremely heartened to hear of adults with spina bifida who were earning their own living, running a home and making a real contribution to the life of the community. Therefore, this section of the chapter tells the story of a young woman who earns her living and runs her own home although she is severely handicapped with spina bifida. No one can tell you more about the day-to-day living difficulties of the disabled than someone who has been battling against them for years.

Anne Grey, who was born with spina bifida cystica twenty-five years ago, has very clear cut views on the subject. She is an excellent person to speak about it as she has obviously thought a great deal about life and has come to terms with the heavy handicap she bears. Her story shows how good training, a practical approach, together with faith in one's self and the better aspects of human nature can overcome problems that may seem insurmountable to the able-bodied onlooker.

Anne Grey has arrived at the point in her life where she can say with pride that she earns her own living, runs her own flat, drives her own car, is a welcoming hostess and is engaged to be married. I visited her in her home after she had returned from work and she told me how things had worked out for her.

She had not been happy at her first school away from home but she afterwards settled in a special school for handicapped children, boarding at first and then later attending as a day pupil. She speaks very highly indeed about what it did for her, and gives it credit for her present ability to be so independent. Anne thinks parents would be unable to push their handicapped child into this state of independence as their urge to help or to make things easier is overwhelmingly strong. Although in her case she had to miss a lot of schooling because of hospital treatments, she got three 'O' levels and acquired a taste for continuing education through reading, which is her favourite pastime.

After her schooling Anne went to a training college to study shorthand and typewriting at a special centre for the physically handicapped where there was also a sheltered workshop. As her parents lived nearby she was able to study as a day student. Later, when she had finished her training, she found it harder than she had expected to get a job and for some time she lived at home with her parents.

For the past four years Anne has been working in a local government office typing planning applications and sometimes typing longhand letters given her by her boss. She heard of this job through an enterprising social worker who went to spy out the land to make sure the office was suitable for Anne's wheelchair before telling her about the job. This social worker found that not only the entrance, the car park, the office, the canteen and the cloakrooms were able to meet the needs, but that Anne could have the job if she passed the tests and felt she could cope with working full office hours.

How on earth, I wondered, did Anne manage to do all that and run a home too? How did she plan her day? She told me:

'Really it's all quite simple if you work it out beforehand. I get myself breakfast at 6.45 a.m. Then I have a bath. I get myself into the bath by easing myself from my chair on to a stool and then into the bath, and I get out and back on to my chair by the same means. Now it's about 7.30 and I switch the wireless on to the news station. If I'm feeling energetic I wash up the breakfast things, if not I leave them till the evening. Then at 7.50 I start making my way out of the flats to drive myself to work in my "Trike". Work starts at 8.30 a.m. The canteen where I have lunch is on the same floor as my office, so I am lucky there. I do most of my shopping at the weekends but if I need something during the week generally one of the other girls will get it for me. At 5.30 I drive myself home. The first thing I do when I get home is to make myself a cup of tea and switch on the wireless.'

Anne told me about her fiancé, John, who is studying accountancy. He too is disabled but not for the same reason, and he is able to walk, though with difficulty. Anne said with some humour, she could beat him easily in her wheelchair if they both set out for the same destination.

It was John, Anne told me, who had pushed her into making the decision to try living on her own and he helped her to find the flat. As he was free during the daytime (it was before his training and he had no job at the time), he went on her behalf to look at a flat he had heard of that they thought would be suitable. To his disappointment that flat had gone but he was told of another, the flat Anne has now. It is run by a housing association that had several different and attractive kinds of housing. Anne regrets that children are not allowed in her area although there are dozens of them in the other sections. Whenever she turns up at the association's launderette to do her washing, she says, it is the children who do it for her.

Anne's parents miss her at home and in particular her mother is still not quite reconciled to her living on her own, but Anne finds they all get along much better now she is independent. She goes home every Monday evening and thoroughly enjoys her evening meal with her parents. She says they are still surprised she is able to live on her own, but she admits they are probably very proud that she can do so.

Living alone for the first time and living in a new area has brought new enjoyments. 'I had never been in a library for instance', Anne said, 'until I lived here. As one of my greatest pleasures is reading I'm delighted to be able to get into a library and to be able to stay there quite a long time and to browse.' Love of reading and love of listening to her radio accounted for the absence of a television set. Her father had offered her one but she had so far resisted the temptation, feeling she could not spare the time to watch television.

For holidays this remarkable young woman likes to go camping under canvas. She goes to a special holiday camp for the disabled. 'When I first heard about it I said to myself "camping with a lot of other disabled people, no thank you". But I tried it and had a marvellous time and so I'm going again this year.'

The camp Anne attends aims at having one able-bodied helper for each disabled person but that seems to be a pipe-dream which cannot be achieved. It is run by various organisations and each leader brings his own helpers from his particular group, which may be the Red Cross, the Guides, or the Scouts, or some other organisation. The campers are not mollycoddled. They have some rough rides struggling through woods and hedges. As Anne says, 'We do just about everything.'

Anne has had what is known in the spina bifida world as 'the bag operation' to deal with her urinary problem. She had to be in hospital for several weeks while it was being performed. She felt apprehensive before she had it done but now is very glad that she did.

It is surprising to hear that, when looking back over her life so far, Anne feels she has had more trouble from pressure sores than she has from her spina bifida. Because of these she had to go into hospital recently. It was then discovered that although she was unaware of it she had a fractured thigh bone, and so had to have a leg amputated. Her doctors told her when she was fully recovered they had been afraid she might not pull through the operation but that it had been quite necessary for her to have it.

I asked Anne what advice she would give to others in her situation and to the parents of spina bifida children. She said:

'Get as much help as you can and don't be afraid to ask for assistance. I recently let myself get ill because I was too proud to ask for help. It was entirely my own fault. Another bit of advice I would give is, don't lock out able-bodied people from your world, you need them! I would say to the younger ones, get the best education you can. I know you may miss a lot of schooling because of treatment, but get the best education your brain will take. You need it more than anyone else because of your physical handicap.'

Anne had advice to give to the parents of handicapped children and that was, 'Don't over-protect your children. It is normal to have a bit of risk in life from time to time and the child who is too protected will never be able to face life on his own.'

To kind, eager, able-bodied would-be helpers, Anne sent this message, 'If you want to help, please see that you know the right help to give! I have nearly been thrown out of this (her wheelchair) by people trying to help.' She tells the story of a disabled man friend who was firmly put back into his car by a bossy passer-by before he could get the helper to realise he had been trying to get out of his car not into it.

'And then', said Anne, 'please, please, don't talk through us, at us or around us. Sometimes one able-bodied person will call to another one in my presence and say, "Does she want a cup of tea?" I find this quite maddening.'

Anne has found there are a good many ways of attracting help if she is in trouble with her car. For instance, living in a block of flats she is lucky in that, if her car seems reluctant to start in the morning, someone always comes and gives her a hand after she has been heard to have a few tries, the sounds of which echo round the central area where she parks. She has found too that if she runs out of petrol or her car gives trouble when she is on the road, she must flash her lights if she wants to be helped and not just sit there waiting hopefully.

In fact Anne Grey is one of those disabled people who manage so well that as an onlooker I found myself forgetting her extra problems in life to the extent of having to pull myself up sharply from time to time and to reflect that this young woman has to plan every movement of her day as though she were working out the moves in a game of chess.

Two other young people with spina bifida who have overcome enormous difficulties, and who have won their independence are the Rushdons. When Mr and Mrs Rushdon were told that the story of their achievements and their experiences in everyday life might give some encouragement to other young people with spina bifida and to the parents of spina bifida children, they were only too willing to co-operate and tell me about themselves and so they invited me to visit them in their home.

They live in a bungalow in Surbiton, a town not far south of London. It is a quiet area of well-tended gardens where in the summer evenings and at weekends the sunshine brings out the inhabitants to mow their lawns, clip their hedges and wash down their cars. The Rushdons are no exception and Victor Rushdon looks after their garden, and the plants in their small conservatory.

The tasks of running the household are divided between them. Denise Rushdon does the housework and the tidying up and most of the cooking. They both do the shopping, Victor doing quite a bit during the week as there is a good fruit and vegetable market near where he works, and Denise doing her share at the weekends, generally on Saturday afternoons since she has to work on Saturday mornings.

Denise has trouble with her balance so she is not able to do jobs like sweeping but apart from this she says there is very little she cannot do. She has a wheelchair which is kept in case of emergency and a metal stick she uses when walking on her own. In fact both the Rushdons can walk without aids in the home but Victor is able to cover far greater distances than Denise. It is easier for him than for Denise and he enjoys it more.

The morning bustle for the Rushdons is very like everyone else's morning bustle except perhaps it is a little more organised. Because Victor goes off first, he gets the breakfast. Denise washes up, tidies up, makes the beds and leaves the house about fifteen minutes after her husband. Then she drives herself to work where she has a special parking place for her invalid car.

Victor does not qualify for an invalid car so he uses public transport to get to work and manages the walk to the bus-stop without any difficulty. He gets home from work about twenty minutes before Denise and so he starts the supper preparations. Naturally they would like to be able to drive about together and so they are saving for a small car.

Denise works full-time as a telephonist for a pharmaceutical firm, a job she enjoys very much, and which she has had for over a year. Victor works for a local authority and has been employed there for about nine years. He has a day a week release from work to study and, having passed his earlier examinations, is in the process of taking his Higher National Certificate in Business Studies (with a bias towards Public Administration). He is, he admits, fairly ambitious. In fact, he says he is much more ambitious now than when he was at school when he saw little point in examinations.

It could be that marriage has made the difference. Seeing that this young couple were obviously so very happy together I asked them how they had met. Smilingly they told me it was a letter on coping with spina bifida that Denise wrote to the ASBAH magazine, *Link*, which had brought them together!

When Denise's letter was published, Victor read it and wrote to her about it. Then they started writing to each other regularly and, after a month or so, decided to meet. Victor visited Denise and her family. They got on so well that time slipped by very fast. So much so that Victor missed his train. Finally, after a scramble he managed to catch the last train home. That first meeting was followed by others and a great number of phone calls. The friendship developed into romance, and engagement and marriage followed. They have now been married for two years.

The Rushdons were interested in the possibilities of having children and discussed the matter with a consultant.

They were told that since they both had spina bifida there would be a 'terrific risk' of them having a spina bifida baby and so they have decided not to have any children, which they regard as a sacrifice in a way but one which they feel is necessary.

Both their lives had been shaped by their education, their training, and the necessary restrictions caused by their handicaps and their periods of hospitalisation. Arrangements have now been made for them to have their hospital check-ups at the same place and at the same time. They both enjoy good general health.

The Rushdons feel that their annual check-ups are very important since both orthopaedic and incontinency problems (particularly prevention of urinary infections) are matters which have constantly to be borne in mind, and they have to have kidney X-rays performed every few years. It is also reassuring for them to know, they say, that their cases are being followed.

Their feelings about education for the young are that every opportunity should be taken to keep the spina bifida child with his intellectual equals although they realise that this is perhaps not possible in every case. On the other hand, Victor pointed out that his eight years at a residential special school helped to create a wish for independence which might not so readily have developed had he attended a day school throughout his education.

Denise and Victor say they have both taught their general practitioners a thing or two about spina bifida in the past and they feel family doctors particularly should be far more informed about it. The Rushdons said the main problem for both of them was incontinence but they both had surgical appliances which dealt with the urinary difficulty. In order to go swimming and wear beach clothes, however, a certain amount of trial and error was needed. Even so they feel this effort is well worth while. Membership of their local ASBAH group, they told me, was an interesting and useful spare time interest since they had both learnt things from it and enjoyed lending a hand to the younger members.

With regard to being a married couple who both have

spina bifida, they said that apart from the fact of not having children, on the credit side they had the assurance that they both understood the difficulties and snags which they encountered in their lives and are able to assist each other to overcome them.

So far as their handicaps were concerned, the Rushdons pointed out that they were less severely disabled than many who had spina bifida. They had been fortunate in that both of them had had the 'closure' operation within a week of being born.

Independence such as that achieved by the Rushdons in difficult circumstances probably owes something at least to their excellent training. Denise attended the Franklin Delano Roosevelt school for the Disabled when she was young, she had one year at Chailey Heritage, and three months at a vocational training centre, where she was trained as a telephonist. Victor started at an ordinary preparatory school, then went to Lord Mayor Treloar College – a special school where he followed a GCE 'O' level course and studied commercial subjects for three years. Unfortunately Denise had had to miss a good deal of schooling while she was having medical treatment.

I asked the Rushdons what they thought about the attitude of the general public. 'On the whole', Victor said, 'people are very, very helpful.' Access to public places is improving but there is still a lot to be done. In their locality, for example, the public library has revolving doors which are unsuitable for wheelchair-users until folded back like ordinary doors. The Rushdons also wished the public were more informed about the condition of spina bifida. To a lot of people, although far more was known now than a few years ago, it still seemed to be a mystery.

Their advice to young people with spina bifida was that they should think seriously about further education, training and what jobs would be available to them. Victor had been so anxious to get a job that he went to his local youth employment officer for the disabled before he had left his school and got the sort of job he wanted within three months of leaving his school. Settling into work had been much easier than he had anticipated. He had had a lot of co-operation from his employers and his workmates.

A feeling of isolation is fairly commonly felt by handicapped people. With Denise and Victor both at work full-time, running their own home and enjoying holidays regularly, I did not think this would be a great problem for them. They have the additional advantage too, of having parents still alive and having brothers and sisters – Denise had a brother and Victor two sisters. They also had nephews and nieces whose company they thoroughly enjoyed.

But they had each known isolation in the past, particularly during holidays from their special schools when their contemporaries at home had formed groups at their schools which did not include them. Denise has memories of not joining the other children when she went to the playing fields near her home and Victor felt that he grew quite apart from the children who had been his friends in childhood. He had certainly felt isolated for a time. Denise had had two years living at home when she had felt very cut off from her contemporaries, but had nevertheless enjoyed the change at the time. Denise and Victor had obviously enjoyed their childhood but were glad the difficulties they and their families had to overcome during these years were over. They now had their own lives and their own home and they could invite other people in to share their contentment. As Victor put it: 'If you can accept the restrictions of your life, you can be very happy.' When I came away from the Rushdons I felt I had been talking to two young people who were finding the greatest possible happiness in their lives together.

Chapter 10

Help from the Specialist Social Worker

One of the people who can be most helpful to families of handicapped children is the specialist social worker. So that I could see some of this work in progress and study many of the children and families, I was invited to go on visits with one who had spent years bringing assistance and hope to dozens of families of spina bifida children, supporting them through painful and difficult times.

The general public has become very much more involved in the situation since she first started in 1960. Very few people had even heard of the malformation in those early days of her work. 'What on earth's that?' parents would ask when they were told their child had 'spina bifida'. Often the mother would ask her, 'Am I the only one?'

This social worker would visit the mother at the earliest possible moment after the birth of her baby, either while the mother was still in hospital or when she had returned home. Usually, at this first visit, the baby had been taken away for its operation. She would talk to the mother about the situation and help her to make plans to deal with the new and quite unexpected circumstances that followed the birth of a baby who had spina bifida.

At an early stage of the conversation she would bring out a file which contained a great many names and addresses. Generally the mother would then ask what was in the file and when told it contained the names and addresses of other parents who had had a spina bifida baby, the mother immediately felt she was not quite so isolated. There were other mothers like her. There were other babies like hers. She was not alone after all.

The social worker would always try to see the father at least once and would generally visit both parents after the first month. In any case she would see the mother again after six months, and every six months from then on. This meant visiting the families in their homes however remotely they might be situated, and travelling in all weathers. It is not surprising she became a very welcome visitor with whom the mothers would discuss personal problems as well as those of their spina bifida baby and other children.

During her visits the social worker would try to explain the nature of the malformation and its possible consequences. She would try to facilitate for the parents the frequent journeys to hospital that were often necessary and she would bring up the matter of possible further pregnancies. The mothers could talk over with her their anxiety that other babies with the malformation might be born to them. She could also help the mother cope with the reactions of relatives and neighbours, the effect on marital harmony and so on.

With her particular devotion to her cause and with the willing co-operation of the medical team, this social worker watched the 'closure' operation performed (not a normal part of her duties). She visited every paediatrician and child clinic in her region. She became so involved she used to haunt the clinic and, to use her own way of putting it, 'lived and dreamed spina bifida'. She did all these things, she told me, so that when parents asked her what was involved in having 'the operation' and other aspects of the problem, she felt she would be able to answer as fully as possible.

Parents whose babies had died were also visited if they wished it but the social worker found that after one or two visits most parents had decided they preferred, if not to forget the matter, at least not to have reminders of their sad loss. On the other hand there were parents who wished to continue the battle with the others, going to meetings and making plans even though their own child had died.

This visiting routine was started several years ago when a survey was started on spina bifida children and their families. (An account of this survey is given in Chapter 13 of this book.) Helped by the social worker and encouraged by her and the medical team, some enterprising parents got together and formed a local branch of the Association for Spina Bifida and Hydrocephalus, an organisation that has given, as it has grown, considerable help to many families of spina bifida and hydrocephalic children all over the kingdom.

Unfortunately not all areas are lucky enough to have a specialised social worker and much more help of this kind is needed. Home visits by a specialist social worker are vitally necessary in order to keep track of the afflicted children and to see the problems of the parents.

Very often, even though the mothers were getting help and advice from neighbours, they were still apt to feel on their own and that they were carrying responsibility of which those around them had no experience. For this reason they especially looked for advice from this social worker, their health visitor and their general practitioner. They became discouraged if these persons did not know of, or showed no special concern for, their child's disabilities.

Sometimes the parents find their difficulties almost overwhelming, particularly when they feel their child is not getting the proper treatment or the right education. If a parent of a handicapped child has really reached rock bottom there is no substitute for the remedy of sending someone kind, experienced and informed to try and sort the situation out.

Chapter 11

Family Stories

The social worker and I visited many spina bifida families by their invitation. Some of the parents and children we talked to are described here so that they can be introduced to other spina bifida families, and to the public who may come to think in terms of children and parents and not just of 'spina bifidas'. Backgrounds, names and so on have been changed, but all the family and home side of the picture is true. The stories have been selected to illustrate different aspects of spina bifida and hydrocephalus.

Achievements with Calipers
As will be seen from the interviews that follow, it often happens that one child or one family is particularly good in some special aspect. Jimmy Green, for instance, one of the first children I visited, had quite a reputation for his sportsmanship and his expertise with his calipers.

The specialist social worker and I arrived at his home before he had got back from school and so we had a chance to talk to his mother with only a younger brother there. This was lucky as it gave the mother a chance to talk about Jimmy. As can be imagined it is quite hard sometimes for the mother to find a chance to have some private conversation about her family life. Banishing the children for too long when the social worker came might make her an unwelcome visitor in the eyes of the children – a reaction to be avoided if possible. Even if the older children are at school, any younger ones around are 'all ears', sometimes discreetly and sometimes very obviously. This is one of the hazards of conversations and interviews with all mothers.

Mrs Green told us that when she was expecting her second child (who is quite normal), she worried so much she almost became resigned to thinking her second one would have spina bifida too. It was only some time after his birth she finally told herself and really believed that 'all was well this time'.

As she was talking about these feelings, the school car drew up outside the house and after a few seconds six-year-old Jimmy Green came striding into the room like a conquering hero. He tripped and laughed, pulled himself up and went to his mother for his greetings kiss. He did indeed manage his calipers with great expertise.

Jimmy's younger brother, David, aged four, came up and gave him a friendly punch which was smartly returned. There was a scuffle and thud and the two boys were struggling on the floor. This went on for a minute or so until order was restored as Mrs Green pointed out to her sons she had visitors.

The younger child was running around and progressing fast and obviously would soon overtake his older brother at least physically. There was certainly some strong rivalry between the boys and the younger one did not yet really understand his brother's problems.

Mrs Green spoke proudly of Jimmy's achievements in fighting his handicap and described how he had striven to master the art of walking with calipers, and dealing with the other physical difficulties in his life. She told me how Jimmy had learned to walk. 'Jimmy just sat there and cried when he first had his calipers on,' said Mrs Green. 'I coaxed him and coaxed him but he still cried. In the end he pulled himself up on the bed. Then he had the rollater frame, then the sticks, and eventually just the calipers. Eighteen months ago he discarded the sticks but he often asks for them back. He liked his sticks. But he's better off without them of course. He mustn't have them back.'

Jimmy has a cheerful disposition. He positively beams. His young brother resembles him. He has a sunny smile too but his is more impish. The two boys get along very well but they have their struggles and Mrs Green has her hands full.

'Sometimes I get aerated and lose my temper, but they're grand really. Jimmy has the valve but this doesn't worry me. He's fallen right on it several times but it's been all right.

'The main difficulty is with his shoes – getting the special shoes made. They take six months to get through. By the time the shoes come they're small and if anything's wrong with them he can't go to school. Then, as you can see, Jimmy's very, very active and he sometimes breaks his calipers. He's very determined to walk. All the children are very determined to walk. Things are moving a lot really towards making life easier. We used to have to attend hospital on different days for different clinics. Now we can combine the visits on one day.'

It is awkward getting Jimmy into the buses but they manage. Mrs Green can reach hospital fairly easily by public transport, and in this she is fortunate. She also enjoys the fact that she is able to do some secretarial work from outside businesses in her home while she is keeping an eye on her children. She finds the spina bifida Local Association a wonderful help and would not consider for a moment missing their meetings. She gets a lot of satisfaction too out of working for another charitable organisation. Even though she has all this to do, she is very aware of the troubles of other families around her and has some time and sympathy to spare for them.

'I get tired because I'm always on the go.' Mrs Green explained this quite cheerfully realising this was the lot of many mothers of young children. She wanted to talk to her visitors quietly but this fact was sensed by the boys and was quite enough to make them curious and reluctant to leave her alone. They wanted drinks of lemonade. They were sent off to get them. They were hungry. They went to get biscuits. They wanted to hug their mother, one each side. This was allowed for a moment or so, then, under their mother's instructions, they went off to 'dial a story' on the telephone, one at a time, a treat they enjoyed daily.

Mrs Green has told Jimmy the simple facts about his handicap. She thought he accepted it, but he did say to the visiting social worker, 'Why can't I walk properly?' He did not complain to his family. 'He has a marvellous personality,' said his mother. 'It's hard, particularly at first. But it all comes gradually. You start to accept it from the beginning. The biggest worry is his incontinence. I worry a lot about that for his future.'

Being told she had a spina bifida baby had not been such a devastating shock at the very beginning, she said, because at first she thought it was just a simple operation. It had not dawned on her at first there was something radically wrong.

'Later I realised it was very serious. Then the social worker called on me and told me there was an Association I could join and that it would help me, and I felt a bit better. When I was in the hospital after Jimmy was born, my father and husband kept coming to see me and I kept thinking my baby had died. Some days after his birth we got to the hospital where the baby was and they said he was coming on very well. That started giving me a bit of hope. Then I saw the social worker again and she helped me a lot. Jimmy was improving all the time. Now we are all at home, Jimmy is six and the health visitor comes to see us every six months. She comes about the younger boy to see how he's doing, but she always asks after Jimmy if he's away at school.'

The Greens have a garden at the back and front of their house and find they have understanding neighbours, but they have been in areas where Jimmy has been teased thoughtlessly. Mr Green has done many jobs of adaptation round the house which have made it easier to run for his wife. He is devoted to his children, but sometimes feels very frustrated on his elder son's behalf.

How a Divorced Mother Manages

Mrs Black is one who has to fight her battles alone or at any rate without the help of a husband, for she is now divorced. Still, she is fortunate in having her mother and her brother's family living nearby.

Her little girl, Jenny, her first child, has spina bifida. She is now six and quite a companion in spite of the fact she is unable to walk and has to get about on a trolley. But Jenny is one of the undaunted in spirit with a smiling face and, like so many of the other children in her situation, she thoroughly enjoys the company of visitors.

Mrs Black, finding herself on her own and being a very sociable person by nature, gets out as much as she can, and when she can make suitable arrangements for her family (Jenny and two younger boys) to be looked after, she likes to go out to work. She needs the money and she needs the outside interest. She has found life very hard without a partner but her children are a great comfort to her. She is determined they will all suffer as little as possible from Jenny's handicap. Her ex-husband, the father of her children, has married again and so does not pay her much money.

Although their difficulties were great during their marriage, Mrs Black says she does not feel having a spina bifida child caused its break-up. She has sadly come to the conclusion that it would have happened anyhow. She has told Jenny everything possible about her handicap and her father's absence from home. Jenny loves both her parents and sees her father occasionally. Like her mother, she is determined to get what she can out of life. She has faced her operations bravely and she takes part spiritedly in whatever is going on whether it is performing at a concert or enjoying communal life at a holiday home. She is lucky at least in that her father is still accessible and that he takes an interest in her and her brothers.

How the Father Helps
The devotion of most of the fathers showed itself in many ways. Many of them worked overtime in order to pay for a family car, holidays or to help meet extra expenses. Many of them had done wonderful conversion jobs in their homes to adapt them to meet the needs of the handicapped child. Many used their skills to make toys and equipment and

many gave up their weekends to take their children sailing, to football matches and to other treats.

Mr Smith was one of the fathers who had shown his dedication to his handicapped son by giving up a very good position and taking up some other work which left him free to have more time at home with his wife and child.

The Smith family live in a pretty, modern house with a sitting room which has a large low window overlooking the back garden. The colours from the flower beds brighten a house that has already been made as warm and welcoming as possible. The low window was one of the reasons the Smiths chose this house, for their son, six-year-old Peter, gets around by propelling himself in his trolley. It is his only means of locomotion on his own. He is very expert with it but of course he is too low down to see through windows placed higher.

Peter was one of the first children in his group to have a trolley and it has made a tremendous difference to his life. Before it came he was a quiet, solemn child. Now, his parents say, he is all 'go'. He goes on errands, opens the front door and goes out to play with the other children. In fact he is so keen on going out to play that instead of having a quiet supper at home, he is given some sandwiches and off he hurries. He gets home from his special school an hour later than the other children and does not want to miss any more playtime.

At the moment Peter has a leg in a plaster cast. He broke it while playing. He came in one day and said casually, 'Mum, my trouser's broken.' That is what it felt like to him, for there was no pain. Although his bones are very brittle, his parents encourage him to get out and about. There are risks in this and it often means trouble for them and for Peter but they all consider the extra benefit of his 'social' life makes it worth while, he so loves parties and calling on people.

Peter often goes to spend a day with his Granny who can manage him well. He loves to do this and he could spend a few nights there too as his Granny is willing and his mother would give it a try, but his father feels more relaxed if Peter is at home where he or his wife can attend to the child during the night if there is any need, particularly as Peter has had nightmares in the past. Still the fact that the Granny is helpful and competent, and that she and her daughter both have the telephone is a great help.

The Smiths are lucky too in that they are able to run a car and they have a garage which Peter finds useful when it is empty. Mr Smith gets home from work in the early evening and can share with his wife the extra complications of running a home and looking after a severely handicapped child who, besides physical help, now needs all the mental stimulation he can get. For Peter has reached the age when everything interests him and he is constantly asking questions. He has recently developed an interest in adult conversation and, like many other children, is not above lurking around the doors, listening and passing on bits of news.

Mrs Smith had a very difficult introduction to the news of her baby's deformity. Nowadays the mother is told as soon as she is considered strong enough after giving birth, but Mrs Smith did not see her baby for many hours. She could get no information from anyone and the only guidance she had was the memory of the anxious glances exchanged by the medical students round her and the sad looks that her husband and father had been unable to hide. Eventually she was shown the baby but he was covered up. She was later told some facts about her spina bifida baby by the doctor and visited by the social worker who did a lot to make her feel she could face her problems.

Mrs Smith was married for several years before she had Peter. When at last she had her first baby and was told he would be very handicapped she said, 'I want him however crippled he will be.' Looking back over the past six years she felt Peter had been a very good baby. 'I was very lucky in that,' she told me. 'I had no difficulty in feeding him, and then he eats well still. He's a glutton with his food in fact. But nowadays I can never really relax with him. I never know what he's up to.'

Peter loves his special school. His vocabulary is excellent but Mrs Smith says she has been told his reading and writing are slow. School gives him something to occupy his mind, a vital necessity to him from now on, and also gives the family a chance to do things outside the home.

Because of their extra restrictions caused by Peter's handicaps the days without school seem very hard to Peter and his parents, especially the long summer holidays, for he has the normal school terms. But he has other interests. He loves being read to, plays chess and he is what his mother calls 'wireless mad'.

Mrs Smith takes a very active part in life apart from looking after her home. She helps her husband with his work and has interests outside her immediate family. She is also lucky in having good friends and neighbours. In fact she moved away from an area where she found the neighbours were unhelpful and lacked understanding.

It takes Mrs Smith an hour to get Peter to bed in the evenings, that is one of the reasons Mr Smith wants to keep him at home at nights. Travelling with Peter is also a major task unless they go in the car and this is not always possible as her husband needs it for business. Mrs Smith can only travel by public transport if someone goes with her for she has the trolley to manage as well as Peter. Peter is very light for his age but he is awkward to move. Soon he will outgrow his trolley and then there will be his wheelchair to cope with. All these problems make visits to hospital or anywhere else a great burden.

Unfortunately the Smiths have some worries outside the home and these Mrs Smith describes as 'worries on top of worries', and they make life harder than it need be. But she would love to increase her family and says she would willingly face all risks.

When she was asked whether having a spina bifida child had brought any difficulties between her husband and herself, she said that it had not.

'But I can't say it's brought us closer together either because there's never been any rift. Obviously it's a great help if you have a religion. Our pastor has been wonderful. I don't know what I'd have done in the early days without his help and support. Of course I worry about Peter and it's a constant worry. He is so frail. But he enjoys life. There are no bullies round here as there were at the other place. And through the Association (ASBAH), and other means, things have improved tremendously in the last six years, and they'll go on improving.'

Some Views on Adoption

Adoption is one of the solutions for families who have had one handicapped child and do not wish to risk having another. I saw that it could be most successful for the adopted child and for the families but some adoptive parents warned of difficulties.

Human nature being what it is, nearly every family has bad moments from time to time and it was useful to hear the views of some of the mothers of handicapped children who had adopted children. Among those I talked to were some who, having decided not to have any more children themselves, had adopted a child and then found they were going to have another baby anyway.

A certain pattern seemed to prevail, particularly if the first baby was the one who had spina bifida. The parents create homes with the idea of starting a family and then, to their sorrow, their baby is born handicapped. They make greater-than-usual efforts to make the home bright, comfortable and easy to run. At first the child occupies the mother pretty well full-time, but as he grows older and takes up less time and attention, the question arises as to whether he should be the only child. Although he may soon go to nursery school which will give the mother a few hours break each day during which she may take a light job, it is unlikely she will return to work full-time unless she is the breadwinner; in that case, of course, a mother-substitute needs to be found for the extra hours she is away.

So on the whole the mother tends to stay in the home much more than the mother of a normal baby. This I think tends to make her yearn for another baby and another chance with a normal child. If the parents find, perhaps after genetic counselling, that the chances of their having another handicapped baby are, in their view, too high, they may after a period of reflection and talking matters over, take steps to adopt a baby. This is, as I have said, often successful but the disadvantages are worth considering.

One is that the adopted child sometimes resents the extra attention given to the handicapped natural child of the parents. Of course this situation arises with the natural siblings too. Another less likely snag is that no one can guarantee anyone is perfect – not even the adoption society.

For example in one family I visited the little girl the parents had adopted developed eczema. The adoption society thought there might be too much work for the young mother to cope with since she already had a spina bifida baby and offered to take the child back, but the warmhearted parents decided to keep her since 'they would certainly have kept her if she had been their own'. The situation is different again when there has been a handicapped child in the family who has died. The gap is very much felt and it is a time for the parents to consider trying to adopt.

Loss of a Severely Handicapped Child

Mrs Field, whose daughter Joan died at the age of three, says she might consider adopting or fostering a child rather than risking having another spina bifida baby.

Joan had been a severely deformed child and she had never been strong. Her mother, who had looked after her devotedly throughout the child's short life, had found much help and comfort from meeting parents in a similar situation to her own. When she met a group of them for the first time, she too suddenly became aware that she and her family were not alone in their plight. Her story may help other spina bifida parents to feel they are not the only ones to have this misfortune fall on them.

Although Joan was very severely handicapped and was often ill during her lifetime and now has died, Mrs Field told those close to her, 'I am grateful to have had her for three years as she brought a lot of love into the family,

especially to me. Joan was so delicate I was aware most of
the time I would probably lose her.'

When Joan came into the world the Fields already had a
son, Bobby, aged three. Joan had been a welcomed baby
though not a planned one. She was born at home. Within an
hour of the birth Mrs Field knew from the nurse that her
baby had a deformity of the spine. She and her husband had
been looking forward to having a little girl, the news was
a devastating blow for them. Mrs Field bravely and stoically
decided she would have to gather her strength and would
'just have to look after her baby more'.

At the time of birth, Mr Field was sent to fetch the
doctor because of the baby's deformity. When he was told
the trouble his first feeling, he said, was one of shock. He
did not know what it all meant or how bad it was, since he
had never heard of the condition before. He was told his
daughter would never be able to use her legs. In spite of
the distress it caused him, Mr Field thinks the doctors were
right to give him the facts in their baby's case, where the
difficulties were to be very great. In fact, the father came
to feel he wanted to know much more about what was going
on.

Within hours of her birth Joan was operated on for
'repair' to her back. When she was six weeks old a Spitz-
Holter valve was inserted. Unfortunately, not long after,
she developed meningitis and had to go back into hospital
to be nursed and to have the valve removed. Joan was left
with severe deformity. Her head became enlarged as a
result of the meningitis and later in her life it became clear
she had suffered brain damage and would be very retarded
mentally. As she grew older and larger her head deformity
was far less noticeable. Because of her original spina bifida
she could never sit or stand and she was incontinent.

Mrs Field had a very gruelling time for the first months
of Joan's life. She had to go to the hospital practically every
day at first and later every two weeks. The journey took
her about thirty-five minutes and she was at the hospital
about one-and-a-half hours. When it came to a matter concerning her own health her doctor was very considerate

and would always call on her if he was needed, never asking her to come to his surgery, to save her that effort at least.

At first Mrs Field felt very nervous when dressing and bathing her baby but later she became quite used to it. She felt the child could never be left alone, but she would willingly leave her with a kind and capable relative for a few hours.

In the months that followed Mrs Field grew to accept but never to be reconciled to her child's handicaps. She became quite expert at managing her daughter, particularly after she had met some other spina bifida families. She was fortunate in having very helpful relatives who would lend a hand and, in due course, she was able to do regular part-time work outside the home. The Fields felt that everything possible was done by the hospital and that, all in all, from medical staff and ordinary people, friends and strangers, they had a lot of consideration.

Mrs Field thinks the other members of her family did not suffer at all from having a handicapped baby in their midst, except that her little boy was jealous of the extra attention the baby got and became more and more demanding himself. Sometimes he was very naughty and difficult. However, he improved as time went by and as he started to go out more on his own. In spite of his jealousy he was fond of the baby and would spend time amusing her.

The Fields' marriage remained a happy one for most of this period although at one time it went through a very bad spell and was really threatened. On the whole Mrs Field found their love for their handicapped child brought them closer together and they considered each other's feelings more than they had before her birth. They no longer took each other for granted. Mrs Field often felt tired during her busy and demanding life. As time went on she felt less depression and anxiety. Her philosophy was, 'You've got to learn to accept things as they are, if you can't accept them, it's very bad.'

During Joan's final illness Mrs Field got very low indeed and became indifferent to most of her other interests and her work. Joan suddenly became much worse. She eventually became semi-conscious, and was taken into hospital. She never regained consciousness, and died after nine days.

Looking back over the three years or so of Joan's life, Mrs Field thinks her worst moment was when Joan got meningitis and had to have her first valve removed. She realises her relatives gave her much more help than they would have done if she had not had a handicapped child. Her husband's life, she feels, was altered very little so far as his work and social life were concerned, although he loved the baby and suffered for her.

She did not find having a handicapped child made her lonely. There was always someone coming or going in her home and although she did go out less after Joan's birth, she was able to do her part-time work most of the time.

Now that Joan is at rest Mrs Field says that although she loved her for those three years, she does feel she would never be able to go through it again, and she would be too afraid of the same thing recurring to attempt to have another baby.

A Girl with Hydrocephalus

In the course of talking to parents of handicapped children it became obvious to me that occasionally one of the parents would dream of an ideal daughter or son, would imagine some young person of considerable physical allure and talent whose only thought was to bring comfort and light to his parents. As we all know if we face the facts, very few parents have this experience in real life even if their children are normal, but such a pipe dream can, on rare occasions, stand in the way of loving the child that exists for his own special qualities.

Some of the ordeals the children and the families have to bear are increased by our ignorance and by our unthinking and inhuman reactions to a child or adult with hydrocephalus. Some of us pride ourselves on our so-called sensitivity, and it is true that the appearance of someone with a larger than normal head often upsets us particularly at a first meeting, but it would be a great step forward if we could cure ourselves of this false feeling and replace it with a genuine sensitivity and reflect the humanity and practicality of those who live and work with this form of abnormality.

I have met many young people with this malformation, young men and women whose chances of being handsome or pretty are small because at the first glance it is clear to the observer their heads are too large and that they have hydrocephalus, and they are isolated.

Rita, a sixteen-year-old girl with this abnormality wore her hair very curly and this certainly helped her to disguise her hydrocephalus. She had several 'O' levels, was first in Latin, French and English at school, and was working hard for her 'A' levels. No one could help being impressed by her courage and her achievements. She was attending a normal school and had some friends there but, sad to relate, she did not meet them out of school. Her best friend was a penfriend, another very intelligent girl who was at university, but she too was having to lead a restricted life because of a heart condition. These two friends found comfort and friendship through their letters to each other and very occasional meetings.

Rita was lucky in having a devoted mother who would sometimes write out her homework, for Rita's hydrocephalus had left her with some lack of co-ordination in her hands. Even so the medical effects of this girl's illness bore no relation to the effects of her deformity on her personal life. They were enough to isolate her from her fellows, which shows the tragedy of 'public' reaction.

For those who make a small effort and befriend such unlucky people, adjustment is made within a few minutes, and the person becomes not a 'hydrocephalic girl' but 'Rita who is good at French'. Rita's two younger brothers were good friends to her. They often teased her but they never teased her about or mentioned the size of her head. However, her mother sadly admitted the brothers were shy of being seen in public with her.

Nowadays, thanks to the valves that can be inserted in the body to draw off the superfluous spinal fluid, this problem will occur less frequently. In the meantime there are many human beings who have to endure and live their lives with enlarged heads through no fault of their own or their family, and it is up to the rest of us to make sure such handicaps are not tragedies.

Better than Normal Homes

One mother of a spina bifida baby girl spoke about the importance of keeping a happy home, but pointed out that doing so required great efforts from the parents. 'When writing and talking about the families of handicapped children', she said, 'there is a great temptation to bring out the normal, or even sometimes better-than-normal qualities of the family and home. But to let the outside world think that such an atmosphere is easily achieved is doing an injustice to the effort and courage of the parents who bring this about.'

Take Mrs Cousins, for instance. Although she is still only in her twenties and is young-looking, she is very motherly and kind. When we called we found a home where everything was shining and clean but with a generous distribution of toys about the place, with some washing airing by the open fire.

The Cousins live in a small stone terraced house that has been newly and attractively decorated and has been adapted by Mr Cousins to suit the needs of their eldest child, Sally, who is eight and has spina bifida. There is a sliding door downstairs between the kitchen and living room and the bathroom too is clear for movements of the handicapped child.

Sally is backward but she is certainly able to learn some things and her mother concentrates in helping her with these. Sally has been at a training centre for four years and, as she was there when the social welfare worker and I called at her home, her mother was able to tell us how her daughter was getting on. 'She dresses and undresses

H

herself like the other children, plays with her brother and little sister, and sometimes quarrels with them. Occasionally she plays up a bit because of her handicap but she's put in her place as the others are. I try to explain to her what we're on about. She understands everything you say to her, that's why my husband says she's not "ineducable". She can learn lots of things.'

During the day, when she is awake, Sally is able to say when she needs the lavatory and to attend to herself, and even during the night she is sometimes able to be continent. She is able to stand for a few minutes without aids of any kind. Mrs Cousins said the medical staff were pleased with her progress and thought she could do without calipers. They had said that she needed to lose some weight, however. At the time of our visit, home and school were asking each other suspiciously who was not sticking to the diet sheet, since Sally was not losing weight as she should have been doing. 'It must be you at home,' one of the teachers had said accusingly to Mrs Cousins! A mystery anyway.

'Sally is a very happy child,' said Mrs Cousins.

'Too contented really. She's lazy in talking. She plays quite happily. She likes the toy car she can ride in. She likes to see other children and play with them and doesn't mind if they get rough. She likes it, rather. But she gets very excited if anybody does anything wrong. She can do quite a lot of things. She can distinguish animals. She liked the holiday caravan. She didn't want to come home from that. Nor did her brother. They both played up because they didn't want to come home and they both got smacked.'

Mrs Cousins said she and her family did go out quite a bit. They went to wherever they could take a wheelchair, places such as the zoo and the park. Sometimes other children would ask, 'Why isn't that little girl walking?' It was upsetting for them. On the other hand Mrs Cousins said everyone 'took' to Sally because she was so pretty.

'And she's had no illness during the past year, only the odd cold. She did have a valve revision two years ago and was in hospital for two or three weeks but she doesn't like hospitals. She doesn't like hospitals at all.'

When asked about routine visits to hospital Mrs Cousins said her husband generally took her there with the other two children. The firm gave her husband the time off for this without deducting any of his money. If she wanted to go anywhere else she put the baby on Sally's wheelchair, which she is not supposed to do but how else, she asked, could she manage? She fits a car-chair for the toddler on the wheel-chair. Mrs Cousins admits she often gets tired but said firmly, 'We have three children and we are very happy with them.'

Loss of a Baby Born with Anencephaly
The Whites too have one of those homes where there is an easy atmosphere and a sense of welcome. However, a year ago they went through the ordeal of losing a new baby because the head was not properly formed. (It was born with anencephaly.) Mrs White's pregnancy seemed quite normal to her. When she was coming to the time when her baby was expected, she went to the hospital with her husband for one of the final check-ups. At that visit she learned the devastating news. She was told by the doctor she was carrying too much water, the baby was very small and the head was not formed properly. She had better come into hospital to have it removed, the sooner the better. She said:

'It was hard to believe at first. The other children are all right and I kept hoping the doctor had made a mistake, though I knew he was right. I had not planned to have this baby but when I found out about it I was very pleased and so was my husband.

'After the baby was taken away I gradually began to feel better. Since I'd been told a week before the baby was born that there was little likelihood of its being alive, it was not too much of a shock, although I was terribly disappointed. I was told within an hour of the birth that the baby was dead.'

Mr and Mrs White already had two healthy, thrustful children, Richard, aged twelve, who is a keen photographer and Jean, aged ten, who has just discovered the joy of reading, much to her parents' relief. These two give their parents a lot of happiness but, like most modern youngsters, they still give plenty of worry too.

Mr White had always been a great child lover. He talked about his reaction at that hospital visit on hearing that the baby they were expecting was probably not living. His words were, 'I felt bewildered more than anything. I did not know what to think when I heard the baby was probably dead. When my wife came out of the doctor's room she was crying, so I had guessed then there was something wrong.'

Later, after the baby had been born, he was asked to call at the hospital to sign the papers. All that, and making arrangements for the baby's burial was part of the sad routine.

Looking back over it all, the Whites feel the hospital advised and treated them well, although they think parents should not have to deal with the burial. Over this matter many parents would disagree.

At the moment Mrs White feels having another baby is too great a risk. She says she might change her mind but does not think on the whole that she will. The stillborn baby has affected her attitude to having further children.

Mr White says his wife does not show her sorrow much to her family. Their daughter sometimes asks why the baby died but that is a question they find difficult to answer. There is still a lot they want to do for their home and life is very busy. They appreciate their good fortune in having had a happy marriage for many years, but Mr White feels it will take some time and a lot of mutual help before they both really get over their loss.

Making Life as Normal as Possible

Perhaps the cases where the youngest child is the handicapped one are the easiest both for the families and the handicapped child. In such cases there are so many helpers around, there is so much the youngest learns from watching his older brothers and sisters, and of course where there are several children in the family the household is a lively organisation and the mother is very occupied.

Mrs May has four children, the youngest of whom, Margaret, aged six, has spina bifida. From the very beginning Mrs May and her husband were determined to make life as normal as possible for their handicapped daughter. They are proud of the fact that she can now walk down their long garden with just her calipers and that she is able to attend a normal school and play a full part in their family life.

Mrs May is a school teacher and it may be that her professional background has considerably helped her in her task of raising a lusty family and at the same time in maintaining the right attitude towards the youngest in these specially difficult circumstances. These might well have resulted in an over-indulged and very spoilt child, all the more so as there is a very helpful and loving granny in the background.

Mrs May takes the view that it is better to face the facts and be prepared if a child is severely handicapped as is the case with her own daughter. She noticed at the time of Margaret's birth, which took place at home, that the baby's feet were not as they should be and she was worried. When the doctor arrived she immediately noticed 'a difference in his manner' from previous such occasions. The doctor told her husband this baby had spina bifida and Mr and Mrs May later faced the situation together. They got over the first shock. What helped, said Mrs May, was that in the first week about half a dozen people came up to her saying they had friends or relatives who had spina bifida babies. She felt less isolated.

The baby, Margaret, was sent to hospital to have the 'closure' operation and later she had the valve insertion. Mr and Mrs May had been told at the beginning there were 'no two alike' and that it was impossible to say at that stage what Margaret's future would be. Certainly in her earliest days she was, as her mother put it, 'almost always in hospital'.

Mrs May expressed her philosophy this way 'You've got to look at the worst that can happen. We've been lucky. The way things have turned out, there is not a lot wrong with her. At six months old she was kicking her legs around like any other baby so I felt sure she would be able to walk. Now at six years of age she gets around very well with her calipers and she plays with the other children. She's not as quick as they are, she can't run, but she wears out her shoes and calipers very fast. She can do everything else that they can do.'

Mrs May said she would not let Margaret miss school at any price. Her daughter had even been to school without boots or calipers when she was waiting for new ones. This policy has paid off. Margaret has an I.Q. that has been assessed as well above average and she is doing well. In the words of her mother: 'She's good at her school work, she sings, she sews beautifully and she enjoys card games. Her granny has helped her there. And she'll have a go at everything in the house, laying the table, washing up or anything.'

Margaret goes to a normal school. She is lucky in having in her vicinity a small village school where there is only one teacher who knows and understands her circumstances. The school is six miles away and she is taken and brought back by car. During the lunch hour she is taken home and assisted in changing by someone who is paid privately to help in this way. The system works very well and she is fully accepted.

Mrs May is hoping to return to her work as a secondary school teacher. She says she has found having a handicapped child a strain, particularly regarding incontinence, although even there the situation is better than they once feared. 'My husband and I thought Margaret did not have any control. She would wet and wet every time you changed her. We concluded she had no control whatever. Over the years however, it does appear to have improved. By the age of six she developed some awareness of her needs.'

Bowel control had been difficult, particularly during the summer. They attempted to rectify this by cutting her down on fruit and solids. Sometimes Margaret was able to go for as long as two hours with no trouble with her bowels so her parents feel things are not too bad. In her mother's words: 'You cannot rely on the bowels at all. But it is not that bad. If it were all that bad we would know where we were. It is just erratic.'

On the good side too is the fact that apart from a short spell when Margaret had a bad chest, she has been free from urinary infection and she has not had to have a urinary diversion. Mrs May was full of praise for her husband's attitude towards all his children 'and so far as Margaret is concerned', she said, 'he is far more patient than I am'.

Of course, many parents would not agree that it was a good idea to 'expect the worst,' as Mrs May suggested. Most parents expressed the view that it was better to wait and see and deal with whatever problem arose.

Rivalry Between Normal and Handicapped Siblings
The fact that one child in a family is handicapped does not prevent the ordinary problems of rivalries and arguments between siblings, as many mothers pointed out to me. The sisters Sandra and Jean Thomas demonstrate this point. Sandra, who is eight, has spina bifida and her sister Jean, who is two years younger, is normal. The two sisters maintain a more or less constant argument which Mrs Thomas thinks both girls enjoy or at any rate find enlivening. She says they fight constantly and will not share their toys.

These disputes go on, she says, because 'sisters are sisters' and not because life is dull or quiet at home. Their baby brother Micky sees to that. He is an extremely robust little boy, not yet two. He is constantly on the go, continually testing for strength various bits of furniture and seems to be shaping up as an international footballer. That, at least, is what his proud grandfather thinks. Judging by the reactions of this youngster's family and small friends (who hide their toys when they know he is coming to play) his training seems well under way. His mother takes all this philosophically, even with a certain amount of pride. She told me that when she last took him to hospital with his sister they were dealt with promptly and encouraged to leave early in case, to use the doctor's words, 'Micky breaks up the fracture clinic'. As can be seen, Mrs Thomas does not have an easy time of it.

The Thomas family also illustrates how a family sometimes choose a home near the school they think right for their children even if the parents would rather be somewhere else. The Thomases live on a modern estate situated on a high hill overlooking the full expanse of the beautiful Rhondda valley in South Wales. Although their home is centrally heated, has very modern equipment and there is everything on the estate that one would think would make a family happy, Mrs Thomas said she would rather be down in the valley, in one of the small stone houses where the rest of her family live because, as she says, 'you cannot stare all day long at a view, however lovely'. Mrs Thomas's in-laws also live on the estate, so she and her husband are not short of company but that Granny too would rather live 'down in the valley' where she came from.

However, Sandra loves her school and Mrs Thomas is afraid that if they moved Sandra would not be so lucky again. Sandra goes to a normal junior school and feels at home not only because she has many friends who are, to use her mother's words, 'wonderful' with her, but because there are one or two other handicapped children there as well to keep her company. The council provides a car to take her to and from school and they have also installed a telephone in the home although Mrs Thomas pays for the calls herself.

Sandra does not miss anything. She goes on trips with the school and with her grandparents. She used to complain about her handicap, saying 'it's not fair' when she saw her younger sister could do so much more than she could, but her family say she has got over that now.

When Sandra first started at school she was very good at her work but her mother says she has found it hard to concentrate lately and she seems to daydream. This may be because Sandra has missed a lot of school recently on account of illnesses such as mumps and influenza, which her friends were having too, and a septic foot and kidney trouble which were due to her special condition. It is not surprising with the absences caused by these troubles that she dropped back in her schoolwork. However at home, her mother says, she does continue her reading and her sums.

Sandra can go upstairs on her bottom unaided, she makes her bed and tidies up and dusts to help her mother. She has had a urinary diversion operation and so wears a special bag that has to be emptied regularly. In common with many children who have spina bifida, she has to have urine tests at regular intervals to ensure she has no kidney infection. She has these tests in hospital and reacts badly to them because, as she told her mother, although they do not hurt her, they frighten her.

Mrs Thomas said she was encouraged by her doctor to have another baby after Sandra's birth. The doctor had said it would be good for her handicapped child. During the pregnancy she became very worried in case the new baby had spina bifida too and she had regretted her decision to have another baby. She worried again about this during her third pregnancy. But she said it was true that the birth of Jean did help Sandra because Sandra made extra efforts to do what her sister was doing.

Mrs Thomas has a lot on her hands but gets strong support from both her husband's family and her own. They have had a hard time financially in the recent past, as her husband was unemployed for two years but now he is back at work. They are happy about this but life is rather difficult since he is on night work. When I interviewed them the whole family had recently enjoyed a week's holiday together in the 'spina bifida' caravan by the sea.

Standing Up to the Rough and Tumble of Life
Sometimes a very handicapped child in a family facing great difficulty such as poverty and unemployment will still

manage to have quite a good time compared with other handicapped children in easier circumstances. Debbie True is very handicapped with spina bifida. She suffers from double incontinence and wears disposable napkins supplied by the National Health Service. She has not had the ileal loop operation as the surgeon did not consider this suitable in her case. Keeping Debbie provided with clothes and bedding is a real problem for her mother since they are very hard up. Mr True is out of work because of an industrial injury.

The Trues live in a council house on a small estate in the midst of beautiful hills. The garden at the back of the house is fully cultivated and every inch of ground is used for growing vegetables. Debbie has two older brothers, both of whom are normal. The oldest boy, aged fifteen, is a keen pigeon fancier and has built a coop for his birds at the end of the garden. He is training to be a cook and he often makes bread and cakes for the family.

Debbie and the boys indulge in fights and struggles of the friendly sort. There are certainly traces of this all round the house but this does not worry Mrs True nowadays, although she admits she is feeling pretty 'low'.

The boys burst home from school during my visit. They were obviously very fond of their mother and their home but they too were very short of clothes and those they have they get through very quickly. On this occasion they had just emerged triumphant from a fight with the lads from the neighbouring village, an annual occurrence I was told. The marauders had come over and broken up the football game. Later these boys will arrange a return raid. It will be a tough fight, they say. This is a fairly lively atmosphere for Debbie to live in and she sticks up for herself. She can make her own way down to the village with her calipers on. She is always asking if she may do this. Her mother says her general health is marvellous. She is able to do quite a lot for herself, like dressing and undressing but she does need her mother's help for toileting.

Mrs True says the boys are marvellous with her and often take her fishing. She has even been camping with them. If they are all arguing Debbie sometimes says to them: 'It's all right for you, you are not a spina bifida. You can walk!'

Debbie is at a special school. Her mother would prefer her to be at an ordinary school if there were one accessible which had adequate facilities for her daughter. As there is no ordinary school place open to her, Debbie attends the special school during the week and comes home at weekends. Her mother says she enjoys it thoroughly. Debbie is tired when she comes home on Fridays but is as right as rain the next day. She is beginning to read and write but is slow with arithmetic. This is not surprising as she has had many interruptions in her schooling.

They play plenty of games in the True household and Debbie also enjoys playing with her dolls and painting. She does not get bullied by the other children in the area. In fact, they enjoy playing with her, especially the younger ones. However, her mother says that if a friend calls with a baby and she makes a fuss of it, Debbie does then get very jealous. Debbie goes away and stays with her cousins sometimes so on the whole she is lucky in meeting and getting along well with so many other children. Her mother says Debbie's being handicapped has not really affected the marriage or affected the pattern of their social life.

Growing Up with Spina Bifida in Canada

Parents with spina bifida children living in areas where the condition is understood and well known and where there are special facilities have considerable advantage over the parents of spina bifida babies in other parts of the world, even where medical facilities are excellent in other respects. Take the case of Mrs March, for example, a girl from southern England whose baby was born in Newfoundland and who now lives near Toronto in Canada. She speaks very highly of her doctor and the specialists she visits from time to time with her son, Stephen, but when she made inquiries about help at a clinic for handicapped children she was greeted with the question: 'Spina bifida? What's that?' She said she felt very cast down and that she was very much on her own.

Mrs March told me about her first baby's birth. She had known she was pregnant when she left England several months earlier. She had a very long labour. As soon as the baby was born she sensed there was something wrong. The doctor attending her recognised the baby had spina bifida and arranged for him to be examined. Within a few hours of birth he had had the 'closure' operation. Mrs March said she felt she had been clubbed on the head when she heard the news of her baby's handicap. She could see her son was very weak. The nuns attending him were anxious to have him christened but Mrs March felt that if she named him she would never get over the loss if he should die, so he was not christened until later when he was in good health. She was told her son would probably never walk. When he developed hydrocephalus Mrs March's mother who had been trained as a nurse, urged her to return to England to see what could be done.

Mrs March flew home with Stephen and, to use Mrs March's words, 'the hydrocephalus seemed to cure itself during the flight'. He never had the shunt operation and there has been no recurrence.

She took Stephen back to Newfoundland and he developed very well. Very soon, when Stephen was only seven months old, Mrs March found she was going to have another baby in spite of the fact that she had been taking birth control measures. Although she had some bad moments of worry about the second child she was glad in a way, she said, that the decision of whether or not to have any more children had been taken out of her hands.

The March's second baby, another boy, was normal. It was not long before another baby was on the way. This time the baby was a girl and she too was normal. Mrs March said she did not worry so much about her third baby, the previous child having shown no signs of spina bifida.

Life for Stephen so far has turned out to be much better than predicted. He is now a fine boy of seven who can walk without aids though he has a limp. One leg is slightly deformed and he is inclined to turn his toes in. His greatest handicap is that he is doubly incontinent. The effects of the hydrocephalus are barely noticeable and, his mother says, are no problem. He looks a handsome child.

Stephen now goes to a normal school in a small town in Ontario. He has many good friends and gets on well with the neighbours. He has been teased verbally by his schoolmates about his incontinence. This has not been easy for him or his family to bear but they have stood up to it well. Stephen gets strong support from his younger brother who, being so near his age, is more like a twin.

Mrs March says people are very kind and easy-going in Canada and she speaks very highly of her doctor. She takes Stephen to see him about once a year and sees other specialists when necessary which has not been often. However, she knows no one else in her town whose child has the same problem and she feels very isolated in this respect. She is very relieved that Stephen, in spite of her earlier fears, is happy and popular and she and her husband feel they have been very fortunate in that the original prognosis that Stephen would never walk has not been fulfilled.

A Family without Spina Bifida

There are very few families without problems even though there may be no handicapped child. When a survey is being done on handicapped children normal children are examined as well to enable as accurate a comparison as possible to be made. The normal children are matched with handicapped children in age, sex and background as far as possible; the normal children are known in research language as 'controls', those with the abnormality that is being investigated as 'index' children.

All the children interviewed and all the case stories so far have been concerned with children with spina bifida, hydrocephalus or anencephaly. This next interview is a talk with the parents of one of the controls, a boy named Trevor Hunter. This control has been picked at random but his story goes to show that everything is not always perfect even for parents of normal children.

Trevor is aged eight and has a younger brother, Peter, aged three. Trevor's health is very good, he takes no medicine and, as one would expect, he never wets or soils. He dresses and undresses himself and washes when told to. He is an affectionate boy who likes to sit on his mother's lap. In this he is unlike his younger brother who has no time for that sort of thing. The brothers are now great friends but they did not have this good relationship until Peter reached the stage where he did not spoil his brother's games.

As Trevor is rather a shy child the parents feel it is good for his morale to have a younger brother around as this means he can show off his superior skills. Trevor's mother is not happy about the school her son is attending at the moment; she prefers the school he went to before they moved, since there 'they really made him work'. At this new school she feels he is allowed to daydream too much. He is not getting good marks. He did well in his IQ tests but is not fulfilling the promise he showed in them. This worries his mother very much. She feels that as he is a quiet and timid boy it is particularly important for him to do well at his school work. He is now in a very low form for his age. At the age of five his parents were told he was eighteen months in advance of his age group. 'I know he can do the work but he's just too lazy,' said his mother. 'In the other school he used to sit near the teacher and every time he raised his head she used to give him a nudge. That was good,' she emphasised. 'He's got to have an education. He's not at all quarrelsome. He's very relaxed. He enjoyed school in the beginning. I don't think he's made any progress at this school. He's gone backwards if anything. He doesn't read at all by himself but he'll read a story for his younger brother.'

It was suggested by the social worker that he ought to have his eyes and ears tested. Trevor had had something wrong with his ears when he was a baby. When asked if he heard the teacher in school Trevor's reply was 'sometimes I do and sometimes I don't'.

Trevor has a five-minute walk to school but, in fact, he has a race with another boy, both to school and back from it, in the afternoon. On the whole he seems to be a 'loner' who prefers television to football and who hates to fight. However, he can punch very hard when he wants to, as his father has found out when playing with him.

When Trevor was younger he was always out with other children. His mother said:

'In the other house he used to play games with the girls who lived round about. They liked him as he was a bit younger than them but up here "it's hit or be hit". Trevor would not do that. He plays with the younger ones until some other boy comes along, then he leaves. He hates gangs and he hates violence so he's not very often with the same age group. He had a lot of pain with his ear when he was a baby so he knows what pain is. But he gets along with his younger brother, although he resented him a lot in the beginning.'

It is perhaps because he is scared of the other boys that Trevor is afraid of the water and will not try to swim with the young boys' club. His father would like to help him here but unfortunately he cannot swim either. (The social worker suggested Trevor should have lessons on his own, perhaps with some relative, since his father cannot swim.)

The central interest of Trevor's life is television. His mother says he has a marvellous memory. He knows all the details about the programmes he watches. He enjoys going to the cinema on Saturday mornings. Trevor also enjoys taking his younger brother out on his bicycle.

'You can't bribe him with anything,' said Mrs Hunter. 'He doesn't seem to want anything. When his Grandad takes him to the seaside he doesn't want to go on the usual things spending money, he'd rather walk by the seashore and look at the pools.'

The family has had several holidays in caravans but

Trevor had never stayed away from home for a long time. Mr and Mrs Hunter often go out and leave the boys with a baby-sitter, generally the grandfather.

Mr Hunter has been off work with a back injury for nearly two years. He is able to do light work and the Hunters run a small car. Naturally Mr Hunter would like to find a suitable job but it would have to be something which did not involve carrying any weight and which allowed him to sit or stand for short periods so that he could ease his back pain. Mrs Hunter suffered from some depression not long ago, it had lasted about twelve months and has now cleared up and she is in very good health.

Chapter 12

Parents' Views and Problems

It is clear that handicaps associated with spina bifida are sometimes very severe and have grave medical, educational and social implications for the child and his whole family. A large number of professional workers are involved in providing the necessary caring services. Do the parents feel they are adequately served by them?

Those I talked to in their homes and at meetings did resent the fact that they had not been properly prepared for the problems they had had to face. Some of them felt they had almost been up against a conspiracy of silence, particularly in the early days.

It is hard to see what kind of preparation would be adequate and the reticence of doctors can well be understood in cases where the medical outlook is very bleak. The fact that accurate prognosis in some cases is very difficult must also be taken into consideration since much depends on the child's reaction to treatment and much is unpredictable.

Then there is the other side of the coin. 'Some doctors paint the picture too black.' These were the words of another parent who had been told his child would never walk but in fact the child is now walking fairly well with the aid of calipers. There is indeed no easy way of telling parents tragic news nor even a way that is correct for all cases. It is a very difficult task for the doctor and one that should never, if possible, be done by anyone inexperienced in spina bifida since a torrent of frantic questions may well follow breaking the news of the baby's handicap.

Another factor much resented was the ignorance of the

general public about spina bifida. Parents felt this ignorance should be dispelled as a preliminary to improving facilities for handicapped people and for changing the whole image of the physically handicapped person. They asked for a book to be written that would 'tell the public and other parents in plain terms what the situation was . . . something we can read through, nothing too technical'. This book was written in response to such requests.

Asked about their problems, many mothers spoke of the day-to-day difficulties of coping with handicapped children. They felt a few simple facts understood and acted upon by the general public and the welfare services could help them a good deal. These are some of the points they mentioned.

Communication between parents and hospital staff seemed to be a bigger problem than the staff realised. Parents said that on the whole they derived comfort and reassurances from regular meetings with the hospital doctor even if nothing had to be done and the only result of their visit was that they were told the child was 'coming along well' or words to that effect. This was even described as a 'tonic' and supports the view that parents and child should be seen regularly.

In times of the greatest stress, such as after a discussion of the need for some further operation, mothers could repeat word for word whole conversations. Of course, their memories might not be perfect but their version of what happened remains imprinted on their minds for a very long time and no doubt becomes reinforced with each recall. It is clear that any ill-chosen words cut deeply. Any sign that the doctor has not understood a difficulty such as, say, fixing the urine bag after a urinary diversion operation, was much resented. Doctor-to-patient language and even tone of voice do therefore need to be taken into account.

Attitudes to students varied. The first intimation one mother had that something was wrong when her baby was born was that she noticed two of the students were in tears. It was some time before she could bring herself to ask what was the matter. Most mothers agreed it was necessary for students to be present at examinations but were very anxious about what the doctors might say about their children to the students.

Quite a number of mothers felt their stress had been increased because there had been no one informed they could talk to while waiting for an operation on their child to be completed though, to be fair to the hospitals, the mothers agreed they had often come before they were asked to or had omitted to telephone beforehand. This criticism highlights the need already mentioned for more specialised social workers who can do much to help the families through such difficult times.

In many cases, even when describing something they thought wrong, parents spoke highly of the hospital staff and were warm in their praises of their particular doctor. Resentment seems to build up as a result of crowded, overtaxed out-patient clinics where parents feel insufficient time is given to their child and where too little explanation is given to parents or is given in language they cannot understand. Many parents told me they thought more should have been said about what was being planned, what was being done and why. Here again a social worker properly briefed could be of help. It is not always enough to state the facts once when the news that is being given is also a shock; in such circumstances it is very hard to take in details. For this reason information may have to be given more than once and explained more fully than would be necessary if the recipient were not so upset.

It was clear that personal expressions of sympathy too are required and expected from the highest medical staff downwards on a person-to-person basis, and lack of them is resented. This may be very difficult for many of the doctors who feel their professionalism would not allow this but, so far as the parents are concerned, this appears to be how most of them feel.

Some mothers say they were never taught how to manage and bath their baby or shown how to cope with his deformities properly. They say they had to find out everything for themselves. This matter is being remedied fast but it is still one of the points brought up by the mothers.

Some minor complaints were made, and perhaps pointing them out may lead to some remedies. A factor no hospital seemed to have considered was the mother's own need for a few moments of freedom and privacy in the lavatory when taking a disabled child to hospital. That she should take the child in with her hardly seems the right answer.

Quite often, too, after a distressing visit to the hospital when doctors, nurses and parents had all had a gruelling time, the parents found they had outstayed such patient amenities as the tea stall and there was no kind of pick-me-up for them before going home which might be many miles away. Perhaps it would be possible for someone such as a 'home help' to be on hand in children's clinics?

Health visitors were criticised for not knowing enough about spina bifida and many of the families said they felt they were doing the teaching. Most of the families were not surprised at the public's ignorance but did resent any sign of it on the part of general practitioners or any officials connected with the welfare services. Even some of the highly qualified medical staff, they said, seemed unaware of some of the day-by-day, hour-by-hour implications for the families of spina bifida babies.

The long waits for special boots and delays over repairs for calipers are the most general cause of frustration and hardship. Several children had missed schooling because they had no boots to wear, and the parents had not wanted their children to go without them. But one determined parent had sent her child to school without them rather than let her daughter miss any lessons. Complaints on this score came pouring out from almost every family and every medical and social worker in the field. It seems we simply do not have anything approaching sufficient resources, or sufficient trained personnel to produce the shoes, boots and appliances needed or to carry out repairs. The difficulty is aggravated by the fact that when it is children who are kept waiting, they have often grown out of the boots and appliances when they do arrive.

Some difficulties arose over transport. There were suggestions that some school drivers were not as helpful as they could be when it came to lifting the children. Perhaps the drivers' duties are not clearly enough defined. There were complaints that some authorities were reluctant to supply escorts and that sometimes transport was provided without adequate strapping to hold the children in place and prevent them from falling. In the midst of these complaints there was a lot of praise for particular schools and particular drivers and authorities. Any failure in the transport system means no schooling for the children, and schooling is a matter of vital importance for them.

Some parents found difficulty in getting other children to come and play, particularly if the child went to a special school and was therefore not 'in' with his local group. One mother described how she had put her severely handicapped child in the front garden with lots of new toys and invited other children in to play. The children came in for a few minutes, looked at the toys and went away, although the handicapped child was very open and friendly by nature. This incident illustrates the emptiness of the long lonely holidays for the children who do not have friends nearby. The goodwill and the warmth of brothers, sisters and family need to be supplemented by friends from outside if possible.

In certain neighbourhoods there were a few isolated cases of bullying or teasing which had the effect of making the handicapped children unwilling to go out to play. The teasing and the isolation I am sure could be alleviated if the parents of able-bodied children would explain matters and set the example, perhaps by inviting the handicapped child into their homes occasionally as happens already in some cases.

The use of certain words such as 'ineducable' caused much pain to the parents, particularly when they knew the child could make advances in social training and in other ways. They interpreted 'ineducable' in many cases as meaning the child could learn absolutely nothing and this made them very despondent and inclined to give up hope.

There were many stories of great kindnesses from friends and neighbours and relatives. There were any number of valiant grandparents who would willingly look after the handicapped child at any time but even they, it seems, sometimes lapsed into spoiling which is forgivable, and 'coddling', which is not.

One mother warned others about the risk of carrying the handicapped child round the house during her work. 'If you do this', she said, 'your baby will always call after you and want to be with you wherever you are. I used to carry my boy round when he was a baby and he was always calling me whenever I left the room for a minute. It took him months to get out of it. Finally he settled for being happy in a doorway swing.'

Some parents suggested it would be useful to have centres where they could be shown what equipment was available and perhaps see examples of the various devices that other families had made and found useful. The Disabled Living Foundation in London does in fact provide such a service, offering country-wide information on aids, appliances, etc., and keeping a permanent display for visitors by appointment.

Most parents thought more of their difficulties of a practical nature should be brought before the public in the hope that someone with a talent for invention might be able to help them. One such difficulty several parents mentioned was coping with a child in a wheelchair at the seaside. Steep hills were an obvious difficulty but one to which they were often accustomed. Getting the wheelchair over pebbly beaches and over sand and sand-dunes was a much harder matter. Anything that made life easier in this respect would be welcomed.

Mothers said the earliest days were the most difficult. If their babies had been taken away for the 'closure' operation they had felt very sad in the hospital wards when they saw the other mothers who had their babies with them. When they returned home they often felt very sensitive about the 'wall of silence' around them because neighbours and even relatives and friends often did not know how to broach the subject of their baby's birth and did not send cards or call, although they did often send flowers. It is difficult to know what should be said in the circumstances and there is probably no formula that would always be right. It does seem, however, that a positive approach and demonstration of interest and helpfulness does mean a lot to the mother who is going through a sad experience, probably not knowing herself how things will turn out for herself and her baby.

One mother described how much better she felt when a neighbour approached saying that she had heard the new baby had spina bifida and asked whether she knew there was another spina bifida baby up the road. 'Suddenly', she said, 'I felt I had not brought a freak into the world after all!'

Again and again parents said they wanted the world to know what their difficulties were, they wanted their children and their problems to be understood. They were particularly anxious that anyone connected with the health and social services who was supposed to assist the families should know at least some basic facts about spina bifida, particularly as it is one of the most prevalent among handicaps today.

Very many of the parents I interviewed belonged to ASBAH and spoke highly of the help they had received from the Association and from the friends they had made through it. There were a few parents however who felt that meeting other parents in a similar situation to their own, and hearing some of the troubles the other children were having, made them very worried in case their own children developed the same problems. However, these parents still wanted to talk over their worries with someone.

This book is based mainly on families in the South Wales area who have had the benefit of support from a specialist social worker well informed on the problems that arise in a family where one of the children has spina bifida or hydrocephalus. Apart from all the practical help and advice she was able to give, I could tell that families derived great comfort from her regular visits. There is a crying need for more such specialists, though it is not always easy to find the right sort of person.

The work requires qualified people of the highest calibre who can act as reliable links between the families and the medical teams, people who are sensitive enough to understand the feelings of the parents and yet practical enough to be able to assist the families in their difficulties, people who are organised enough to keep accurate records, people who can drive a car and find their way about the countryside in all weathers and go into every sort of home. It helps, I believe, if the worker in this field has had a family of her own.

It can be seen from all this that the work is demanding. On the other hand it is deeply satisfying for the person who feels in sympathy with the families and wants to help those who carry extra burdens. It is work that is of constant interest from the medical, psychological, sociological and humanitarian point of view. The worker is a member of the team and it is a marvellous job for the right, dedicated person.

Chapter 13

The South Wales Investigation

Certain communities seem to have a greater susceptibility than others to producing offspring with malformations of the central nervous system. Because it is probable that certain environmental factors act as trigger mechanisms, an investigation was started in 1960 centred on the agricultural Vale of Glamorgan and the mining valleys of Glamorgan and Monmouthshire, an area in which the spina bifida incidence is the highest reported in any population that has been studied. Furthermore, the incidence there for anencephaly was exceeded only by that in the Northern Ireland series of Stevenson and Warnock (1959). The overall incidence of the three malformations in the South Wales area was 8·100 per 1,000 births. (Carter, David and Laurence, 1968.) The investigation is still continuing and will not be completed for several years.

The investigating team sought to establish the incidence of the malformations and whether there was any relation between the incidence and geological background, water supply, rainfall, sunshine, population density, distribution as to town and country areas and other factors. Some of the findings are given below.

There was no obvious relationship between the local incidence of abnormalities and the occurrence of any type of rock formation. Nor did there appear to be any relationship between the type of water supplied and the incidence of the malformations, nor did rainfall seem an important factor. Nothing could be said about the effect of sunshine as information was incomplete. There was an unduly high proportion of mothers over forty among those who gave

K

birth to babies with one of the three conditions mentioned. A clear majority of the spina bifida and anencephaly babies were first-born. The father's age did not appear to have any significant effect. Blood groups did not offer any clues since no significant difference in this respect was found to exist between mothers of spina bifida babies and the general population.

A family study to ascertain the mode of inheritance and to get accurate information about the recurrence risks was part of the investigation. (Carter, David and Laurence, 1968.) It was found, as was expected, that there was a considerable concentration of sibships (brotherly or sisterly relationships), with some families having as many as four cases.

There seemed a higher than expected incidence of these malformations among the mother's maternal cousins but this was not definite. There was shown to be a higher incidence in the mother's sister's children than in the mother's brother's children. It was thought that this conclusion should be studied further since it was not found in the control series. It suggests a special maternal influence. The investigation did not show that the mother who had already had a large family was more likely to have an affected baby. Social class and seasonal effects in this series were judged to be insignificant.

Another aspect examined was consanguinity. There was no indication that consanguinity was the cause of the high rate of spina bifida in this area.

As spina bifida was such a large problem in South Wales it was felt that the repercussions of the malformations on the family and the community should be investigated in depth as they were largely unknown. An investigating team consisting of two psychiatrists, E. H. Hare and K. Rawnsley, a reader in applied genetics, K. M. Laurence, a research social worker, Helly Payne, an educational psychologist, B. J. Tew and a research teacher, E. R. Laurence, carried out a survey and based it on 126 families in which a child with spina bifida, anencephaly or uncomplicated hydrocephalus had been born in South Wales between 1964 and 1966.

Control families were selected on the basis of sex of the index child, his position in the family, social class and area of residence. The social worker visited the mothers soon after the birth of the baby and thereafter at six-monthly intervals, except in cases where the baby had died and the parents did not wish to have any more visits. No mother refused the first interview. Eight cases were later dropped from the survey because of refused interviews, and in three cases the family moved from the area.

When the children reached the age of five they were assessed by the educational psychologist, and the research teacher followed this up by visiting the schools where the children were placed. The reports based on this survey are part of a continuing study of the children, following them into primary school, secondary school and onwards.

When a mother bears an obviously malformed child severe emotional distress is bound to be in store for herself and her husband. The study tried to assess this stress and the help that was necessary in these circumstances.

The psychological problems caused by frequent hospital visits, worry about the possibility of another pregnancy, uncertainty about contraceptive measures, and the fears of parents who wanted more children but were concerned about the risk of another child being affected in the same way, were examined.

Replies from the parents showed that fathers were more distressed than mothers by the first news of their child's deformity; but it became clear that the mothers, at the time of the first interview, had not really taken in the situation. For instance one mother, who was partly under the anaesthetic when told her baby had spina bifida, said it took her a long time to realise the nurses and doctor were talking about her baby in particular and not about all babies of that kind.

At the second interview, one month later, parents were asked whether they thought a mother should be told about the baby's condition at once or later. Ninety out of ninety-nine mothers thought the mother should be told at once but thirty-three out of ninety-six fathers thought the mother should be told later either by the father or at the same time as the father. The reason put forward for telling the mother later was that the mother was not in a fit state to take things in immediately after the birth. But one of the drawbacks of any delay was that it might give rise to false hopes and exaggerated fears.

Parents were asked at this interview how they felt about the way the news had been broken to them. Eighty per cent thought it had been done in as kindly a way as possible, 8 per cent had some reservations and 12 per cent thought it had not been done well. Among the criticisms was one from a mother who had felt the doctor was shouting at her but such a memory might well reflect the tensions of doctor and mother at this extremely difficult moment.

This study also considered the reactions of relatives and neighbours. It had been thought that parents might often have been hurt by stupid or thoughtless remarks from relations and neighbours but in fact such incidents were rare. Most parents said they did not mind people knowing of the baby's condition and that friends and relatives had all been sympathetic and helpful. One father whose baby, his first, had spina bifida cystica, said he tried to avoid people in the beginning but as the neighbours gradually realised what had happened they were so very kind he felt he could go into any house and everybody would show sympathetic under-standing. Another parent, a mother aged seventeen whose first baby had spina bifida cystica, said that no one made unkind remarks but that one of her very close relatives liked to show people the baby's back. The young mother did resent this but was too shy to say anything.

The report found that parents did have to face the remarks of relatives, and perhaps their own thoughts, on whether it would have been better if the baby had died. Almost every mother, it states, wanted her baby to live, especially when she had had it at home and looked after it. The impression received was that mothers were anxious and unsettled while the baby was in hospital for surgical treatment, and happier when they had the baby home, and this was true even when the baby was obviously in a poor state. Mothers continued to love and to want their babies even when they were badly deformed.

Some parents did not at first want their baby to live, when told what the future might hold. But after a month they wanted everything possible to be done to save the child.

The report told of one family where a mother aged twenty-one and a father aged twenty-four had a spina bifida cystica baby with severe hydrocephalus. The father said when he saw the baby he wished they would not continue to keep the child alive, if the future was to be as bad as they had painted it. But he was surprised how concerned everybody was and how good and kind they were. The mother said all she wanted was to see and have her baby.

Another couple where both the parents were aged seventeen gave birth to a spina bifida baby, their first child. The mother had been told that the baby was never likely to walk. At the first interview she said she would much rather the baby died, as if the child were a cripple she would not know how to look after her. The father intervened with the remark: 'She doesn't love the baby yet as she should; she hasn't handled her much, but she'll come to it.' At the six-month interview the mother was reported to be 'terribly fond of her baby'.

One pair of parents pointed out that it was better to see the baby first before coming to any decisions. 'Before seeing him', they said, 'everything seemed vague to us and a terrifying picture was painted. Later we got quite a different picture from what the doctor said.'

One father described his feelings of anger that the birth of a spina bifida baby should happen to them. He had felt completely out of patience with everybody. Neither he nor his parents had ever heard of 'spina bifida'. He could not believe it had happened.

Another father spoke of his relief when told there was no known cause but that it was neither the fault of his wife nor himself. A mother said she had not wanted to get to love her baby too much in case she lost it.

Regarding the effect on marital harmony of having a spina bifida cystica baby, the report found that the emotional and physical strain of having and caring for a malformed child was likely to influence marital harmony in a way that reflected the depth of affection between the parents and the maturity of their personalities.

In the great majority of cases, and whether the child survived or not, parents said that the event had brought them closer together. In only one case had the baby been neglected by both parents and had had to be taken into care of the children's department. There were three cases in which the mother's preoccupation with the child or the father's inability to accept it had led to quarrels and separations. (It should perhaps be pointed out here that family feeling is very strong in Wales and such cohesion might not apply in other areas such as large cities where the rejection of handicapped children seems more common.)

Parents were asked at the interviews whether they felt they had been given enough help and advice by the hospital, their family doctor and their health visitor. A third of the fathers and more than half the mothers felt they could have been given more help and advice.

These parents appeared to feel, not so much that they should have been given more instruction, but that the doctor or nurse did not seem to appreciate what worries and anxieties the parents had to bear and did not say the simple words of comfort which would have shown their understanding and sympathy.

At interviews which took place after one year the parents were asked about their visits to hospitals. Their children nearly always needed observation or treatment which meant either stays in hospital or hospital visits. Of twenty-three mothers whose children were living at one year, only four received partial assistance from the ambulance service for journeys to hospital; six went by car, the rest by bus or train. Fourteen mothers visited hospital at least weekly during the first three months. The cost of journeys varied from 'negligible', where the mother went in the family car, to about one pound or so when the mother went by train with a relative. The cost of these journeys was paid by the families and some husbands said they worked overtime to earn the extra money. The time taken by the journey each way varied from ten minutes to two hours, averaging about an hour, and the average time spent at the hospital was about an hour and a half. This had meant that a visit to hospital tended to occupy a large part of a day.

Another subject on which questions were asked during this study was the matter of risk for further children. Mothers were asked whether their child's condition had affected their attitude to having further children, whether they thought there was a risk it might happen again, and whether anyone had told them about such a risk.

At the one-month interview a third of the mothers said they would definitely not want any more children, and one-fifth said they would be cautious. These proportions were somewhat less at the six-month interview.

One-quarter of the mothers said they thought there was no risk that the same trouble would happen to them again and one-quarter did not know whether there was a risk or not. Of the mothers who thought there was some risk the majority (two-thirds) either did not know how great it might be or assessed it as 'small'. When asked whether anyone had talked to them about a risk, 60 per cent of the mothers said 'no' at the one-month interview and the proportion was the same at six months. Of those told about a risk by their doctors the general impression the mothers got was that the risk was small. Parents said they had been told: 'it could not happen again', 'there was a one-in-a-million chance', 'one chance in 50,000', 'extremely unlikely', 'a slight chance'.

One mother aged seventeen, whose first baby, a spina bifida cystica, had died after four days told the interviewer: 'My doctor said it was a bit of bad luck and there was no likelihood of it happening again.' She wanted another baby and was not trying to avoid pregnancy but said she would be very afraid in case it went wrong again. (Clearly these opinions that the risk was small do not accord with the views of the risks given by geneticists which are based on family studies.)

The authors of the report in their discussion point out that their information was obtained largely from parents who, under the stress of emotion, may have misunderstood some of what was told them by doctors and nurses. They also point out that where parents express dissatisfaction with the way their case was managed this may in part be due to the psychological process by which feelings of anxiety or guilt are converted into expressions of hostility and blame.

The authors considered that the question of when parents should be told of an abnormal birth and how much should be said of its nature and causes had to be decided by the doctor or nurse from their experience and from their assessment of the particular circumstances.

When it came to breaking the news to the mother the authors felt it would be wiser to break the news to her only in the most general terms at first and leave more precise explanations till later, perhaps when the husband could also be present.

It was pointed out that when considering the welfare of families with a severely handicapped child the presence of other stresses must be taken into account. The emotional strain of accepting the abnormality, the anxieties of nursing a delicate or fretful child and the wearing effect of frequent hospital visits are common to most of such families. Further problems such as ill-health of the parents, the needs of other small children in the family, a father's unemployment, bad housing or living with uncongenial in-laws, might all increase the natural burden, while neurotic traits or immaturity of personality of one or both parents might increase it beyond endurance.

The team also considered the following aspect of the problem. Help is sought from many different departments of the hospitals, several departments of the local authority and perhaps from voluntary organisations too. In the hospitals a large number of specialists are likely to be involved: obstetricians, paediatricians, neuro-surgeons, urologists, geneticists, psychologists, physiotherapists and social workers among others. Conflicting advice can be given and result in confusion.

The authors concluded that most benefit would result if

one person, a worker with special experience in the field, were to act as co-ordinator for the provision of social and medical help to each such family over an appropriate area. He or she would be a person with close knowledge of the problems in each family and to whom the parents could turn for advice. They thought too there was a strong case for special hospital centres to provide major surgical and orthopaedic treatment for all cases within an appropriate region.

The necessity for genetic counselling was emphasised. Other studies had established that when a mother had had one child with spina bifida cystica or anencephaly, the risk of recurrence was undoubtedly a serious one. The recurrence rate had been found to be one in thirty-three in Birmingham (Record and McKeown, 1950), one in seventeen in Rhode Island, USA (Macmahon *et al*, 1953), one in eighteen in Southampton (Williamson, 1965) and one in sixteen in Sheffield (Lorber, 1965). In South Wales where the study was being made the recurrence rate after a spina bifida birth was one in fifteen and after an anencephalic birth, one in twenty-five. (Data taken from report made in 1966.)

The authors said that in advising parents they would have to consider how far a realistic statement of the recurrence risk might lead to undue anxiety; yet in general and particularly where parents asked for information, the doctor should quote the best evidence from medical studies or else refer the parents to a clinic for genetic counselling. If on the basis of this advice the parents decided they wanted to avoid further pregnancies then there were good reasons why contraceptive advice and means should be made available to them. Good contraceptive methods, by relieving a mother of her fear of another pregnancy with its attendant risk, was an important factor in marital harmony. A period without further pregnancy would give the parents time to become accustomed to the strains and future problems of bringing up a handicapped child and so enable them to take a measured decision on having further children.

Investigation of spina bifida cystica and family stress is of particular interest here since it makes known the effect of spina bifida on the whole family and shows that the repercussions may be very great and that every means possible should be used to see that the family is not dragged down by them.

Many further studies have been carried out, based on the South Wales investigation. Some of these have indicated that the original view taken, that spina bifida children have normally distributed intelligence, was too optimistic. For instance, a study published in 1972 showed that there was a significant difference in the distribution of intelligence between the control group of children and the index group, and that this was because of brain damage. Many other aspects have been under review and as more is learnt about children with spina bifida it becomes easier to find what will help them and the families most.

Chapter 14

Future Prospects

The investigations and work carried out on spina bifida in South Wales have attracted a good deal of attention, as indeed has work done in Sheffield, Liverpool, Edinburgh, Northern Ireland and other centres in the United Kingdom. That in itself has helped to educate the public about the extent and seriousness of the problem and the needs of the families and the needs of the children. This is all part of a general increasing awareness of the requirements of the handicapped, particularly in respect of their being able to use all public buildings.

More sophisticated devices, some controlled electronically, may come into use in the not too distant future to help people with spina bifida. Power-assisted splints and calipers may be able to assist walking and other movements. A greater degree of help may come with the development of electronic devices for bladder control though unfortunately it does not seem likely that it will be possible, in the foreseeable future, to give to the spinal cord those functions which have never been there.

With the use of amniocentesis on women who are especially at risk, followed by the possibility of selective abortion where indicated at the end of the twentieth week, as mentioned in Chapter 2, there may well be a small reduction in the incidence of spina bifida in the near future. In the hope of making a greater reduction, a test is being developed which may be carried out on the mother's blood at about the fifth month and is capable of being used on all pregnancies. If this test proves not to miss too many abnormal babies and at the same time not to call in question too many normal pregnancies, it could be carried out routinely along with all the other tests normally carried out during the ante-natal period. It will, however, be a year or so before any large-scale trials are complete and it can be decided whether this test will be feasible as a matter of routine. This approach, however, must always be regarded as second best and it is hoped that one day it will be possible to discover what causes these malformations.

It seems we can also expect a more scientific method of detecting which babies are likely to do well. It was shown, for instance, in papers published in 1973[1] that clinical features present at birth can give useful data for predicting the baby's chances for life in terms of mobility, intelligence, continence and overall disability, and also for his risks of death caused by renal failure. It was indicated that the fundamental question of achieving a reasonable degree of independence is governed almost entirely by the neurological deficit.

In a paper published in 1974 exploring the effects of operating wherever possible on babies with spina bifida cystica, and pursuing an aggressive surgical approach to the abnormality, its author estimated 'that in the United Kingdom alone, with an incidence of 2·5 cases of spina bifida per 1,000 births, each year about 500 additional families would have to cope with a severely handicapped surviving child'.[2] The question of which babies should be operated on is one doctors have been considering for some years and one in which they are increasingly concerned.[3] Much is being published about it in the medical journals and the titles of some of the papers describing these important studies on this subject are included in the list at the back of this book.

The best hope of all would be to find out what triggers off spina bifida. Much research is going on in this sphere

[1] Hunt, G., Lewin, W., Gleave, J., Gairdner, D., 'Predictive factors in open myelomeningocele with special reference to sensory level', *B.M.J.*, *4* (1973), pp. 197–201.

[2] Laurence, K. M., 'The effect of early surgery for spina bifida cystica on survival and quality of life', *Lancet* (23.12.74), pp. 301–4.

[3] Lorber, J., 'Early results of selective treatment of spina bifida cystica', *B.M.J.*, *4* (1973), pp. 201–4.

too. For instance, folic acid deficiency may possibly be a cause. Many factors which from time to time have been under suspicion have proved not to be important. Blighted potatoes, for example, were thought at one time to have been a cause of spina bifida, but further work suggests these are not the important factors they were first thought to be, as was pointed out in Chapter 2. However, sooner or later the causes will probably be identified and real progress can then be expected in finding a method of prevention.

In the meantime most of the children and the parents battle on bravely. True, they are occasionally brought very low, sometimes to the point where trouble seems to follow on trouble and life no longer seems to hold any pleasure. The few cases where the mother has been left to manage with a handicapped child on her own are particularly distressing, but all families with a handicapped child carry a much heavier burden than the rest of the community. There is great need for support and understanding from everyone, from the strangers who pass by on shopping trips and who give a kindly greeting, to the closest relatives and friends who may be able to take on some regular commitment to help the parents. The children and their families ought to be given all necessary backing so that they can enjoy their days and play as full a part as possible in the life of the community. Then perhaps they may become what they long to be, just ordinary happy families.

Glossary

amniocentesis: Technique of getting amniotic fluid from the uterine cavity.

anencephaly: Condition in which the head of the baby is not developed properly.

calipers: Metal supports for legs.

cystica: Cystlike.

encephalocele: A lump on the back of the head or neck, usually covered by skin, containing meninges and often brain tissue.

hydrocephalus: Greek term for 'water on the brain'.

ileal loop: Transplanted piece of intestine into which the ureters are transplanted to act as an artificial bladder.

lesion: Area of damage.

meninges: Membranes enveloping brain and spinal cord.

meningocele: Condition where the meninges only form the cyst-like protrusion.

myelomeningocele: Condition where meninges and spinal cord tissue form the abnormality.

meningitis: Inflammation of the brain or spinal cord.

occulta: Hidden.

orthotist: Appliance-maker.

parapodia: Supports to aid in movement and standing.

spina bifida: Literally, 'spine split in two'.

solonaceous alkaloids: Substances found in the potato when it is exposed to sunlight. The substance is responsible for a bitter taste.

sphincter: Muscle serving to open or close an opening tube.

stoma: Outlet fashioned by the surgeon for collecting the urine in a bag or other receptacle from the artificial bladder.

ureter: Duct by which urine passes from the kidney to the bladder.

Selected Bibliography

Carter, C. O., David, P. A. and Laurence, K. M., 'A family study of central nervous system malformations in South Wales', *Journal of Medical Genetics* (1968), *5*, pp. 81–106.

Emanuel, I. and Sever, L. E., 'Questions concerning the possible association of potatoes and neural-tube defects, and an alternative hypothesis relating to maternal growth and development', *Teratology*, *8*, No. 3 (December 1973).

Hare, E. H., Laurence, K. M., Payne, H. and Rawnsley, K., 'Spina Bifida and family stress', *British Medical Journal* (1966), *ii*, pp. 757–60.

Hare, E. H., Payne, H., Laurence, K. M. and Rawnsley, K., 'The effect of severe stress on the Maudsley Personality Inventory in normal subjects', *British Journal of Social and Clinical Psychology* (1972), *11*, pp. 353–8.

Hunt, G., Lewin, W., Gleave, J. and Gairdner, D., 'Predictive factors in open myelomeningocele with special reference to sensory level', *British Medical Journal* (1973), *4*, pp. 197–201.

Hunt, G., 'Implications of the Treatment of Myelomeningocele for the Child and his Family', *Lancet* (8.12.73).

Laurence, E. R., 'Spina Bifida children in school: preliminary report', *Developmental Medicine and Child Neurology*, *13* (1971), Supplement No. 25, 'Hydrocephalus and Spina Bifida', pp. 44–6.

Laurence, K. M., 'The Effect of Early Surgery for Spina Bifida Cystica on Survival and Quality of Life', *Lancet* (23.12.74), pp. 301–4.

Laurence, K. M., 'Early pre-natal screening for foetal malformations and abnormalities', *Lancet*, 1974. In press.

Laurence, K. M., Carter, C. O. and David, P. A., 'The Major central nervous system malformations in South Wales, i. Incidence, local variations and geographical factors', *British Journal of Preventive and Social Medicine* (1968), *22*, pp. 146–60.

Laurence, K. M., Carter, C. O. and David, P. A., 'The major

central nervous system malformations in South Wales. ii. Pregnancy factors, seasonal variations and social class effects', *British Journal of Preventive and Social Medicine* (1968), *22*, pp. 212–22.

Laurence, K. M., and Tew, B. J., 'The natural history of Spina Bifida Cystica and Cranium Bifidum Cysticum: the central nervous system malformations in South Wales', Part IV, *Archives of Diseases in Childhood* (1971), *46*, pp. 328–38.

Lorber, J., 'Early Results of Selective Treatment of Spina Bifida Cystica', *British Medical Journal* (1973), *4*, pp. 201–4.

Renwick, J. H., 'Hypothesis: Anencephaly and Spina Bifida are usually preventable by avoidance of a specific but unidentified substance present in certain potato tubers', *British Journal of Preventive and Social Medicine* (1972), *26*, pp. 67–88.

Tew, B. J. and Laurence, K. M., 'The ability and attainments of Spina Bifida patients born in South Wales between 1956 and 1962', Developmental Medicine and Child Neurology (1972), *14*, Supplement No. 27, 'Studies in Hydrocephalus and Spina Bifida', pp. 124–31.

Tew, B. J. and Laurence, K. M., 'Mothers, brothers and sisters of Spina Bifida patients', *Developmental Medicine and Child Neurology* (1973), Supplement 29, 'Studies in Hydrocephalus and Spina Bifida', pp. 69–76.

WHO, Public Health Papers (42), 'The Prevention of perinatal morbidity and mortality'.

Zachary, R. B., 'Ethical and social aspects of treatment of Spina Bifida', *Lancet* (1968), *11*, p. 274.

Appendixes

Appendices

Appendix I

THE ASSOCIATION FOR SPINA BIFIDA AND HYDROCEPHALUS
(ASBAH)

A Company Limited by Guarantee

Devonshire Street House, 30 Devonshire Street
London W1N 2EB
Telephone: 01-486 6100
          01-935 9060

There are Local Associations in the following places (Spring 1974). Addresses of the Honorary Secretaries can be obtained from the National Office.

ENGLAND

Blackpool and Fylde
Bolton and Bury
Bournemouth, Christchurch and District
Bristol
Bromley
Buckinghamshire
Burnley
Cannock and Walsall
Chesterfield
Consett and District
Darlington and District
Derby
Devon and Cornwall
Don and Dearne
Dudley and Wolverhampton
East Anglian
Essex
Gloucester North
Greenwich
Halifax and District
Hampshire-North, West Surrey and Berkshire
Hampshire-South
Herts. and South Beds.
Huddersfield
Hull and District

Isle of Wight
Jersey
Kent
Leeds and District
Leicestershire
Leigh and District
Lincoln
Lincolnshire
Liverpool
London:
  Barnet Area
  Ealing Area
  North East (Forest) Area
London South
Lunesdale (Lancaster)
Manchester and District
Mansfield, Worksop and District
North Beds. and Northants.
North-East (Northumberland)
Nottingham and District
Preston
Rochdale
St Helens and District
Salisbury and District
Sheffield
Southampton and District
Spenborough (Yorks.)

Staffordshire
Staines, Hounslow and District
Stockport
Surrey (NASBAH)
Sussex
Swindon and District
Teesside
Trafford (Manchester)
Warrington and District
Warwickshire
Wessex
Wigan and Chorley
Wirral
Worcestershire
York

WALES
Mid-Wales and Border Counties

North Wales
South Wales

NORTHERN IRELAND
Ballymena
Belfast
Lurgan and Portadown
Mid-Ulster

There is an Association in
SCOTLAND
7 South East Circus Place,
    Edinburgh EH3 6TJ
and one in EIRE
c/o Mrs Kinsella, 66 Martello
    Hill, Carrick Estate,
    Portmarnock, Co. Dublin

GRANTS MADE AS PART OF ASBAH'S RESEARCH PROGRAMME

Research into causes		£
Manchester University	Cell structure of the central nervous system	3,494
Sheffield University	Towards work in the Pathology Department	3,700
	Quantimet electronic scanner for the Congenital Anomalies Research Unit	14,500
Research into hydrocephalus		
Queen Mary's Hospital, Carshalton	Research into the colonisation of the valve	2,400
Westminster Children's Hospital	Electrical impulses of the brain	5,000
Royal Infirmary, Hull	High frequency recording apparatus	4,300
Pre-natal diagnosis of spina bifida & anencephaly		
University of Edinburgh	Chemical analysis of amniotic fluid	4,500
Research into social & intellectual consequences of spina bifida & hydrocephalus		

		£
Sheffield Department of Child Health	Study into the care of the spina bifida child and support of the family	2,240
Welsh School of Architecture	Suitability of schools for the physically handicapped	1,070
Sheffield University	Aptitudes of school leavers with spina bifida cystica/hydrocephalus	7,000
	This work is now being continued as a service to adolescent patients	10,000
Hospital for Sick Children, Great Ormond Street	Correlation of spina bifida and hydrocephalus with ocular abnormalities	500

The Association hopes to raise £60,000 to fund a Spina Bifida Research Fellowship.

Appendix II

1. *This list combines some of the special boarding schools, boarding homes and establishments for the further education and training of the physically handicapped and delicate that accept cases of spina bifida.*

Board of Managers, The Children's Convalescent Home and School, Meols Drive, West Kirby, Cheshire

Board of Governors, Lord Mayor Treloar College, Froyle, Alton, Hampshire

Board of Governors, Florence Treloar School, Holybourne, near Alton, Hampshire

Board of Governors, Holly Bank School, Halifax Road, Huddersfield, Yorkshire

Board of Governors, Mossbrook, Cinder Hill Lane, Sheffield 8, Yorkshire

Boys' and Girls' Welfare Society, Bethesda Special School, Schools Hill, Cheadle, Cheshire

Central Council for the Disabled, Hesley Hall School for Seriously Disabled Children, Tickhill, Nottinghamshire

Chailey Heritage Hospital and School, Chailey, Sussex

Dr Barnardo's Homes, Ian Tetley Memorial Home and School, Killingham, Yorkshire

Dr Barnardo's Homes, Princess Margaret School, Middleway, Taunton, Somerset

Dr Barnardo's Homes, Warlies School, Waltham Abbey, Essex

English Congregation of the Dominican Sisters, St Rose's Roman Catholic School, Stroud, Gloucestershire

Gateshead Board of Managers, The Cedars School for Physically Handicapped Children, Lowfell, Gateshead, Durham

Kent Board of Managers, Valence School, Westerham, Kent

Lancashire Board of Managers, Singleton Hall School, Poulton le Fylde, Lancashire

Liverpool Board of Managers, Abbots Lea School, Beaconsfield Road, Liverpool 25, Lancashire

Liverpool Board of Managers, Children's Rest School of Recovery, Greenbank Lane, Liverpool, Lancashire

Manchester Board of Managers, The Margaret Barclay Residential School for Crippled Children, Moberley, Cheshire

National Children's Home and School, Chipping Norton, Oxfordshire

National Children's Home, Elmfield School, Harpenden, Hertfordshire

Nottinghamshire Board of Managers, Thieves Wood School, Near Mansfield, Nottinghamshire

Queen Mary's Hospital School, Carshalton, Surrey

Shaftesbury Society, Burton Hill House School, Malmesbury, Wiltshire

Shaftesbury Society, The Victoria School, 12 Lindsay Road, Branksome Park, Poole, Dorset

Shaftesbury Society: Hinwick Hall School, Nr. Wellingborough, Bedfordshire

Shaftesbury Society, Trueloves School, Ingatestone, Essex

Staffordshire Board of Managers, Wightwick Hall Special School, Tinacre Hill, Compton, Staffordshire

Yorkshire N.R. Board of Managers, Welburn Hall School, Kirbymoorside, Yorkshire

GREATER LONDON AREA

Church of England Children's Society, Halliwick School for Physically Handicapped Girls, Winchmore Hill

Dr Barnardo's Homes, John Capel Hanbury House School, Garden City, Woodford Bridge

Hillingdon Board of Managers, St Michael's School, Hoel Street, Eastcote, Pinner

Shaftesbury Society, Coney Hill School, Hayes, Kent

WALES

Glamorgan Board of Managers, Glamorgan Residential School for Physically Handicapped Children, Erw'r Delyn, Penarth.

Joint Committee of North Wales Authorities, Gogarth School, Llandudno

There are also many Special Day Schools that accept children with spina bifida. Information about them can be obtained from the Department of Education and Science.

2. *Residential sheltered employment (voluntary organisations)*

Barrowmore Village Settlement, Chester
Dorincourt Industries, Leatherhead, Surrey
Enham-Alamein Village Settlement, Andover, Hants.
John Groom's Association for the Disabled, Edgware
Papworth Village Settlement, Cambridge
Portland Training College, Mansfield, Notts.
Red Cross House, Largs, Scotland
School of Stitchery, Great Bookham, Surrey
St Loye's College, Exeter
Yateley Textiles, Camberley, Surrey

3. Training colleges for the disabled

Derwen Training Centre, Oswestry
Portland Training College, Mansfield, Notts.
Queen Elizabeth's Training College, Leatherhead, Surrey
St Loye's College, Exeter

4. Residential welfare homes and workshops

Ashley House Home for Physically Handicapped Boys, Bognor
    Regis, Sussex
Enham-Alamein Village Settlement, Andover, Hants.
John Groom's Association for the Disabled, Edgware
Papworth Village Settlement, Cambridge
Red Cross Centre, Largs, Scotland (Occupation Centre and Work
    Centre)
School of Stitchery, Great Bookham, Surrey
Searchlight Workshops, Newhaven, Sussex
Woodlarks Workshop, Farnham, Surrey

5. Organisations concerned with further education and assessment

Dene Park (Spastics Society), Tonbridge, Kent
Hethersett Vocational Guidance Centre, Reigate, Surrey (Royal
    National Institute for the Blind)
Sherrards Industrial Rehabilitation Unit (Spastics Society), Welwyn
    Garden City, Herts.
Star Centre for Youth, Ullenwood Manor, Cheltenham, Glos.
    (Further Education Centre)
Wolfson Comprehensive Assessment Centre, Bloomsbury

6. Research Centre

National Bureau for Co-operation in Child Care, Fitzroy Square,
    Bloomsbury

Appendix III

SOURCES OF RESEARCH FUNDS

1. Voluntary bodies in the United Kingdom

ASBAH (Association for Spina Bifida and Hydrocephalus), Devonshire Street House, 30 Devonshire Street, London W1N 2EB

Tenovus, 111 Cathedral Road, Cardiff, Wales

The Children's Research Fund, 6 Castle Street, Liverpool 2

The Mental Health Research Fund, 38 Wigmore Street, London W1

The National Fund for Research into Crippling Diseases, Vincent House, Vincent Square, London SW1

The National Society for Mentally Handicapped Children, 86 Newman Street, London W1

The Nuffield Foundation, Nuffield Lodge, Regent's Park, London NW1

2. National and Voluntary Bodies in the United States of America

Association for the Aid of Crippled Children, 345 East 46th Street, New York, NY

The National Foundation (March of Dimes), 800 Second Avenue, New York, NY 10017 (More than 3,000 local chapters)

The National Institute of Neurological Disease and Stroke, National Institutes of Health, Bethesda, Maryland, 20014

Index